TRAILS OF CENTRAL ARKANSAS

Legend for Maps

This page provides a brief guide to using this book. Trail descriptions contain:

Trail Name → Oak Savannah Trail

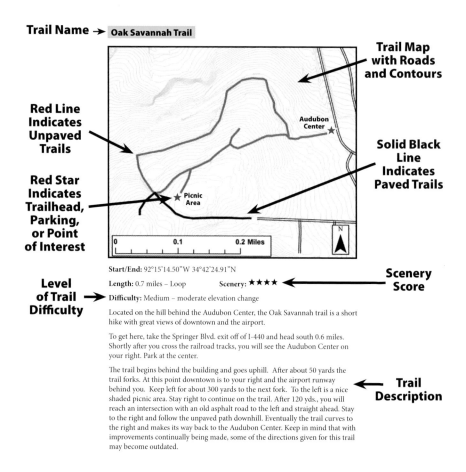

Trail Map with Roads and Contours

Red Line Indicates Unpaved Trails

Solid Black Line Indicates Paved Trails

Red Star Indicates Trailhead, Parking, or Point of Interest

Audubon Center

★ Picnic Area

0   0.1   0.2 Miles

N

Start/End: 92°15'14.50"W 34°42'24.91"N

Length: 0.7 miles – Loop   **Scenery:** ★★★★ ← **Scenery Score**

Level of Trail Difficulty → **Difficulty:** Medium – moderate elevation change

Located on the hill behind the Audubon Center, the Oak Savannah trail is a short hike with great views of downtown and the airport.

To get here, take the Springer Blvd. exit off of I-440 and head south 0.6 miles. Shortly after you cross the railroad tracks, you will see the Audubon Center on your right. Park at the center.

The trail begins behind the building and goes uphill. After about 50 yards the trail forks. At this point downtown is to your right and the airport runway behind you. Keep left for about 300 yards to the next fork. To the left is a nice shaded picnic area. Stay right to continue on the trail. After 120 yds., you will reach an intersection with an old asphalt road to the left and straight ahead. Stay to the right and follow the unpaved path downhill. Eventually the trail curves to the right and makes its way back to the Audubon Center. Keep in mind that with improvements continually being made, some of the directions given for this trail may become outdated. ← **Trail Description**

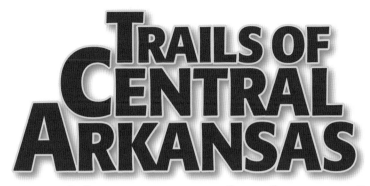

TRAILS OF CENTRAL ARKANSAS

A Guide to Central Arkansas' Land and Water Trails

HIKE, BIKE, PADDLE

BY JOHNNIE CHAMBERLIN

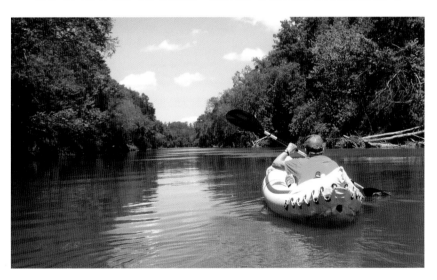

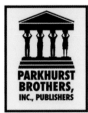

PARKHURST
BROTHERS,
INC., PUBLISHERS

Little Rock, Arkansas

www.parkhurstbrothers.com

Parkhurst Brothers books are distributed to the trade through Chicago Distribution Center, phone 800-621-2736. Copies of this and other Parkhurst Brothers, Inc., Publishers titles are available to organizations and corporations for purchase in quantity by contacting Special Sales Department at our home office location, listed on our web site.

Printed in the United States of America

First Edition, 2012

12 11 10 9 8 7 6 5 4 3 2 1

For Library of Congress Cataloging date, consult publisher web site after publication date.:

ISBN: 978-1-935166-89-4

Book design and cover design: Harvill Ross Studios Ltd., North Little Rock, AR

Acquired for Parkhurst Brothers, Inc., Publishers by: Ted Parkhurst

Editor: Sandie Williams

All maps and photos are by Johnnie Chamberlin.

This book is dedicated to Pops.
Thanks for going on that 18 mile hike in August with me.

Acknowledgments

This book never would have happened if it weren't for my dad and our use of his Tim Ernst books. He and his dad got me into hiking, backpacking, and boating.

Warnings

Most of the trips mentioned in this book can be completed in one day but hikers should take adequate water, food and first-aid supplies. As with any hike into the wilderness, a person should be alert to the presence of insects, snakes and poisonous foliage and always respect "No Trespassing" signs.

Table of Contents

Introduction

I got the idea to write my first book, Trails of Little Rock, after working for Audubon Arkansas where, as part of my job, I walked along all the major creeks in Little Rock and the surrounding area. I also spent many days floating Fourche Creek performing assessments, searching for rare plants, planting trees, and clearing log jams. On and off the job, I came across numerous trails that I'd never heard about and most people I told about them had never heard of them either, so I decided to put them all in a book.

This book serves as kind of a second edition to that book, but covers a larger area so North Little Rock, Bryant, Conway, Jacksonville, Cabot and other Central Arkansas communities don't feel left out. All trails in this book are still within a 45 minute drive of Little Rock and most are much closer.

It is my hope that people using this book will become as passionate about trails and greenspace as I am and will encourage their elected officials and neighborhood associations to create more interconnected trails that serve as viable transportation routes in addition to providing wonderful recreational opportunities.

This book is not exhaustive but it contains information on dozens of great hikes, floats, and bike and pedestrian trails in Central Arkansas.

If you know of any trails I missed, feel free to e-mail me at johnnie.chamberlin@gmail.com and I will include it in any future editions of the book and credit you

Map of Trails

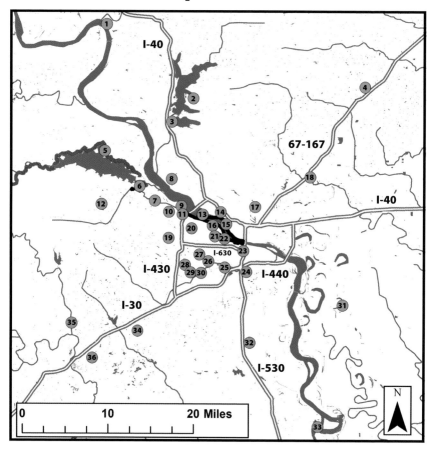

1. Cadron Settlement
2. Camp Robinson Special Use Area
3. Bell Slough
4. Lonoke County Regional Park
5. Ouachita Trail
6. Pinnacle Mountain State Park
7. Little Maumelle
8. Lake Willastein
9. Two Rivers Park
10. Conner Park
11. River Mountain Park
12. Section 13 Park

13. Pfeiffer Loop
14. Burns Park
15. Emerald Park
16. River Trail
17. Five Mile Creek
18. Dupree Park
19. Rock Creek Trail
20. Reservoir Park
21. Allsopp Park
22. Knoop Park
23. Macarthur Park
24. Audubon Center
25. Fourche Creek
26. Coleman Creek Greenway

27. Boyle Park
28. Brodie Creek Upstream
29. Brodie Creek Park
30. Hindman Park
31. Toltec Mounds State Park
32. Lorance Creek Natural Area
33. White Bluff Trail
34. Mills Park
35. Saline River
36. Tyndall Park

Trails Organized by Difficulty

Trails by Region

Top 10s

Top 10 Most Scenic Trails

1. Pinnacle Mountain East Summit Trail 84
2. Emerald Park 56
3. Pinnacle Mountain West Summit Trail 86
4. Little Maumelle 136
5. River Trail 100
6. Fourche Creek Middle Section 132
7. Brodie Creek Upstream of Col. Glenn 40
8. River Mountain Park 98
9. Knoop Loop 62
10. North Fork–Steel Bridge Rd. to Lyle Park 144

Top 10 Trails for Kids

1. Lake Willastein - Maumelle 64
2. River Trail 100
3. Paved Loop Trail -Two Rivers Park 124
4. Kingfisher Trail at Pinnacle Mountain 90
5. Boyle Park Bike/Pedestrian Trails 28
6. Pinnacle Mountain West Summit 86
7. Dupree Park 54
8. Allsopp Park South 18
9. Little Maumelle 136
10. Knoop Loop 62

Top 10 Trails for Solitude

1. Section 13 Trails 112
2. Brodie Creek Park to Hindman 42
3. Fourche Creek Upper Section 130
4. Lorance Creek Natural Area. 68
5. Fourche Creek Middle Section 132
6. Boyle Park West Outer Trail 36
7. Nun Trail–Boyle Park 32
8. North Nature Trail–Boyle Park 34
9. Quarry Trail Pinnacle Mountain 94
10. River Mountain Park 98

Foot and Bike Trails

Allsopp Park

Allsopp Park covers two valleys located between the Hillcrest and Riverdale neighborhoods of Little Rock. The park includes numerous dirt trails through the woods as well as some improved/paved ones that are used by bikers and hikers.

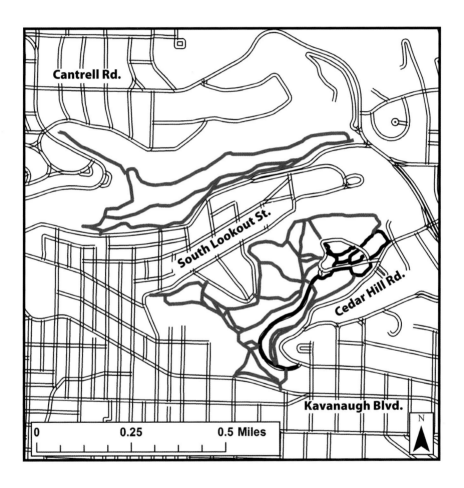

Allsopp Park – North

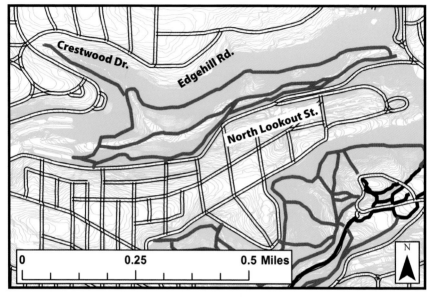

Start: 34°45'57.44"N 92°18'53.47"W

Length: 1.5 miles – Loop   **Scenery:** ★★★

Difficulty: Moderate – Sometimes steep with roots and rocks on the trail.

The main entrance to this trail is at the intersection of Cantrell and Allsopp Park Rd. There are more entrances along Lookout Rd and behind some apartments. This section of Allsopp consists of three trails that run roughly parallel to each other while following a creek channel. In general the most well worn trail is the middle trail, which follows a sewer right of way in several places. The most scenic trail is probably the northern route since it is the farthest from busy roads and the highest in elevation.

There's a small parking lot located at the main entrance and if you begin your journey here and stay to the right, you will be on the most scenic branch of the trail. The first 100 yards of the trail is rather steep and then levels out for most of the next 0.75 miles. The trail has a couple of small bridges that cross streams which can become raging waterfalls during heavy rains. At the fork in the trail going left will lead down to the middle trail. Taking the trail on the right will follow along Lookout and will eventually lead back to the parking lot.

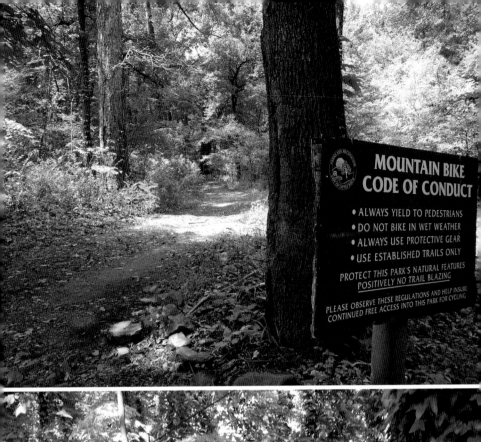

MOUNTAIN BIKE CODE OF CONDUCT

- ALWAYS YIELD TO PEDESTRIANS
- DO NOT BIKE IN WET WEATHER
- ALWAYS USE PROTECTIVE GEAR
- USE ESTABLISHED TRAILS ONLY

PROTECT THIS PARK'S NATURAL FEATURES
POSITIVELY NO TRAIL BLAZING

PLEASE OBSERVE THESE REGULATIONS AND HELP INSURE
CONTINUED FREE ACCESS INTO THIS PARK FOR CYCLING

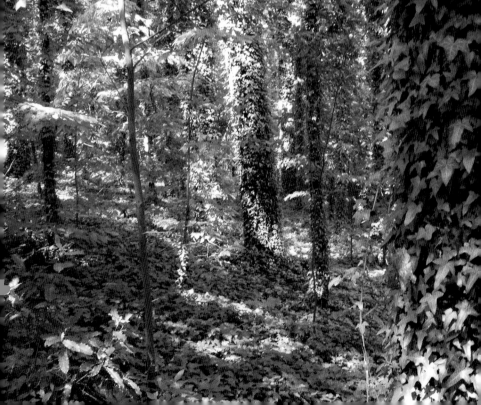

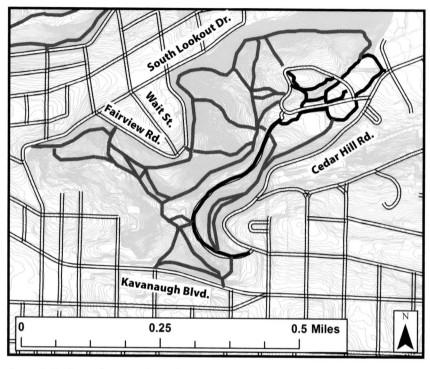

Start: 34°45'43.54"N 92°18'52.86"W

Length: 1.8 miles – Loop   **Scenery:** ★★★★

Difficulty: Moderate – Sometimes steep with roots and rocks on the trail.

With over three miles of trail packed into this 80-90 acre park, there are plenty of trails to explore. The map isn't inclusive since there are multiple forks and less worn trails in the area, but I think that I've represented all the major trails and intersections. Unless you live in the area, the easiest place to access these trails is by entering Allsopp Park from Cedar Hill Road and parking near the tennis courts or baseball field. Other entrances are located along Kavanaugh, Beechwood, Fairview Rd, and in the parking lot behind Pulaski Heights Baptist Church. The trails are scenic and may, at times, contain quirky bits. When I explored this area, I came across a small cedar tree that had been decorated as a Christmas tree. In many sections of this trail it's easy to forget you are in the middle of a city.

This hike starts at the parking lot near the tennis courts. Take the paved trail on the right, next to the creek. After 100 yards, turn left onto the dirt trail and head up the hill. The trail is somewhat steep for the next 100 yards and then levels out. Stay right for the next 1300 yards. As you near the Fairview entrance you will see an interesting rock garden covered in moss. From there head south and again stay right. You will pass a tall concrete structure covered in graffiti. Then cross a creek, and pass another similar concrete structure. At this point giving good directions becomes difficult as there are several intersections. From the second concrete structure, head south and stay on the more prominent trails. This will take you to a section of trail paralleling the Promenade on Kavanaugh. After passing the two Promenade entrances, follow the trail to the right which runs behind the church. Turn left onto the paved trail and head downhill for about 150 feet before turning right onto another dirt trail. If you are tired of rough trails at this point, stay on the paved trail and follow it for about 880 yards back to your car. Otherwise, stay right on the dirt trail for about 525 yards and you will come to a grassy area near the baseball field. If you head toward the playground and tennis court you will return to the parking lot and your car.

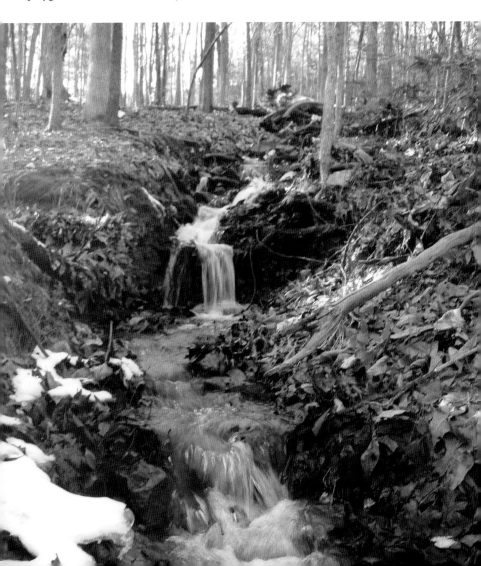

Audubon Nature Center

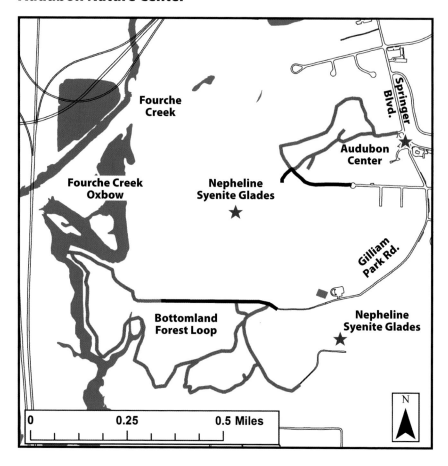

The Audubon Arkansas Nature Center, a 400+ acre natural area located near downtown Little Rock, is home to a wide variety of habitats including: willow oak flats, bottomland hardwood forest, oak savanna, upland pine/white oak forest, rare nepheline syenite glades, and a cypress oxbow. This book describes three trails at the center, but more are being built all the time.

For more information visit the center at 4500 Springer Blvd. or go online to ar.audubon.org.

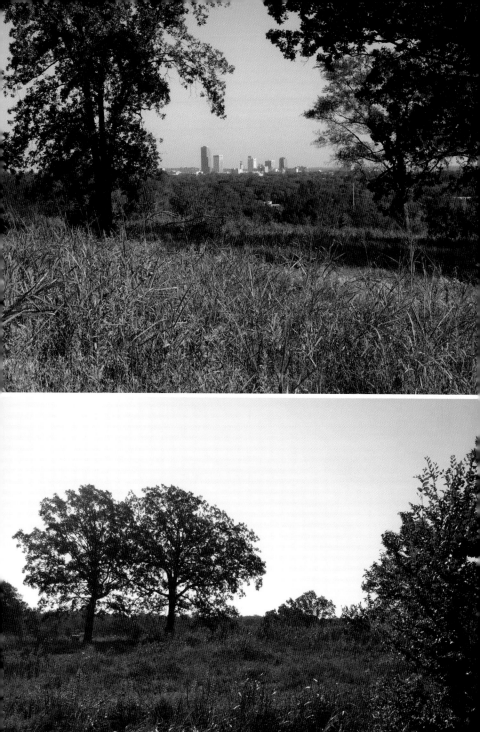

Oak Savannah Trail

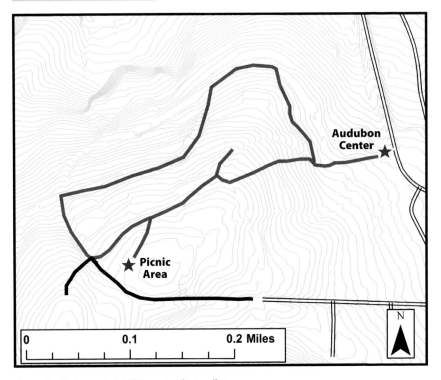

Start/End: 92°15'14.50"W 34°42'24.91"N

Length: 0.7 miles – Loop   **Scenery:** ★★★★

Difficulty: Moderate – moderate elevation change

Located on the hill behind the Audubon Center, the Oak Savannah trail is a short hike with great views of downtown and the airport.

To get here, take the Springer Blvd. exit off of I-440 and head south 0.6 miles. Shortly after you cross the railroad tracks, you will see the Audubon Center on your right. Park at the center.

The trail begins behind the building and goes uphill. After about 50 yards the trail forks. At this point downtown is to your right and the airport runway behind you. Keep left for about 300 yards to the next fork. To the left is a nice shaded picnic area. Stay right to continue on the trail. After 120 yds., you will reach an intersection with an old asphalt road to the left and straight ahead. Stay to the right and follow the unpaved path downhill. Eventually the trail curves to the right and makes its way back to the Audubon Center. Keep in mind that with improvements continually being made, some of the directions given for this trail may become outdated.

Bottomland Forest and Oxbow Loop

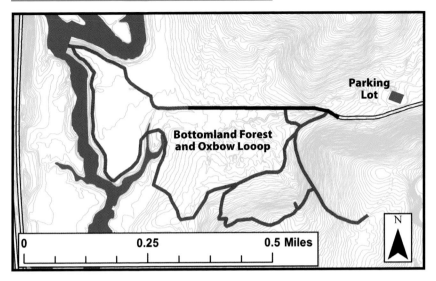

Start/End: 92°15'36.12"W 34°42'1.92"N

Length: 1.6 miles – Loop   **Scenery:** ★★★✦

Difficulty: Easy – flat, paved or gravel in places

Starting from the parking lot, head west past the metal gate and down the old paved road. Going counter-clockwise around this trail makes it easier to follow and takes you through the least scenic section first, thus saving the best for later. You will pass a gravel road heading off to your left and a dirt trail to the left just a little farther down the road.

After about 500 yards, the road switches from asphalt to gravel. The trail winds through a bottomland hardwood forest and along an oxbow of Fourche Creek for the next 1,300 yards. Along the way the gravel ends and gives way to a dirt trail. After walking along the edge of the cypress-lined lake for a while, the trail heads back into the woods. When you come to the power line right-of-way, be sure to head straight and find the trail instead of following the power line right-of-way.

The next 500 yards leads through a wooded area. The Uplands Loop Trail heads of to the right. If you are ready to go back to the parking lot, stay to the left and then turn left on the gravel road and you will pass a stone pavilion on your right before reaching the paved road.

Uplands Loop

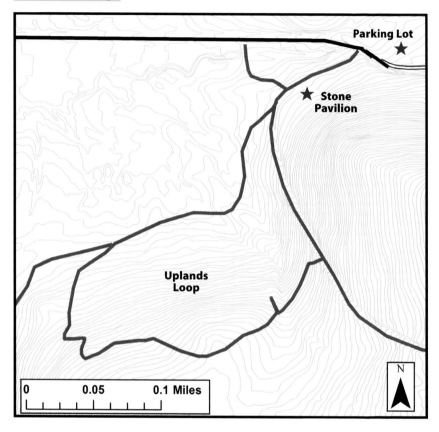

Start/End: 92°15'36.933"W 34°42'1.515"N

Length: 0.6 miles – Loop   **Scenery:** ★★★

Difficulty: Moderate – moderate elevation change, rocky in places

This is a fairly new trail and is pretty rocky in places with a lot of muscadine, pine, white oaks, and poison ivy growing along the trail.

From the stone pavilion head south down the gravel road. Follow the gravel road past the metal gate and up the hill. After about 250 yards turn right on the small trail which branches off the gravel road. If you reach a fence you've come too far.

About 100 yards after the gravel road, the trail will split. To the right is a short spur to a bench and wildlife observation area and the main trail is to the left and uphill. After about 350 yards the trail levels out and is rough in places. At the bottom of the hill the trail converges with the Bottomland Forest and Oxbow Loop. Keep left to extend the hike along the oxbow or turn right to return to the parking lot.

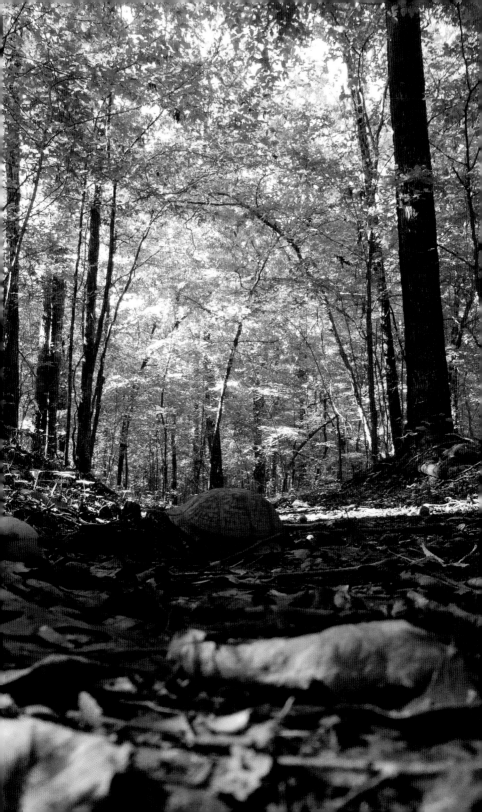

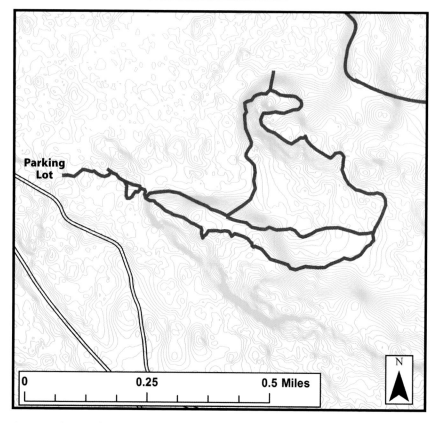

Start/End: 34°56'20.73"N 92°25'3.94"W

Length: 2.25 miles – Loop   **Scenery:** ★★★✦

Difficulty: Easy – Mostly flat or slight incline, crushed gravel

Bell Slough WMA covers 2,000 acres near Mayflower, just east of I-40. The parking area is located off Grassy Lake Rd., about half a mile east of Hwy. 365, about two miles south of the Mayflower exit. The trail is fairly flat and has several wildlife observation platforms.

The sign at the trailhead mentions that parts of the trail can be accessed by wheelchair but are "moderately challenging."

From the parking area the 5'-6' wide crushed gravel trail heads east. After 150 yards, you will reach a blind by a pond off to the left. Shortly after that the trail forks briefly. Where the trails come together, there is a large open waterfowl rest area off to the north that is closed part of the year. Head south to stay on the main trail and soon you'll reach a 4-way intersection. Take a left. This area is home to lots of mayapples and buckeyes. Over the next 300 yards, look for cacti

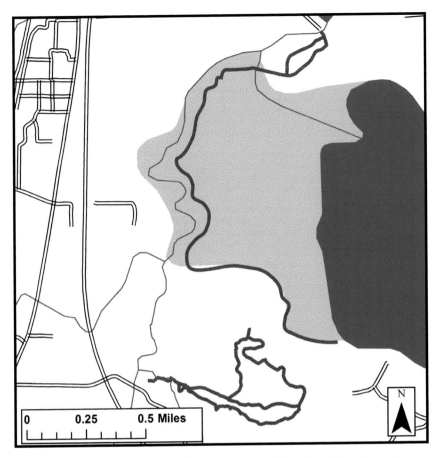

0   0.25   0.5 Miles

and redbud underneath willow oaks, sweet gum, red maple, white ash, and post oaks. At the fork, take a left and head downhill. In 600 yards the trail forks again. A short distance to the left is a photo blind. The main trail continues to the right and heads uphill through a drier area with cedars, blackjack oaks, and more cacti.

In 600 more yards you will reach another fork. Both ways take you back to the parking area. The trail to the right follows a small creek for a bit before reaching familiar territory. Head straight at the fork for better views. After 700 yards, you will reach some benches near a ridge with some views. From there it is 200 yards back to the big intersection, where you just follow the trail you took in to get back to your car.

Another trail enters Bell Slough just off Dam Rd. and almost connects to this one. That other trail follows the levee and is sometimes under water. Maps and more information can be found at http://www.agfc.com

Boyle Park

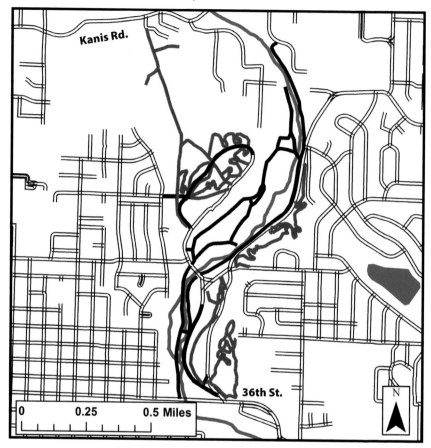

Located between Col. Glenn. Rd., University Ave. and Kanis, with Rock Creek flowing through its center, Boyle Park is a large urban park with over 10 miles of both paved and unpaved trails. Many of these trails run along Rock Creek or side streams and ponds, providing access to fishing and good birding. The paved trails are well-maintained, fairly level, and excellent places for parents to take their small children or strollers. The dirt trails are typically much steeper and more rugged. They are used primarily by mountain bikers and hikers. If you visit the park be sure to notice the interesting clump of tupelo trees right at the car bridge across Rock Creek.

The two trails referred to in Trails of Little Rock as "Archwood Winding Trail" and "Southern Ridge Trail" now have official signs labeling them as "North Nature Trail" and "South Nature Trail" respectively and these new titles are used on the pages that follow.

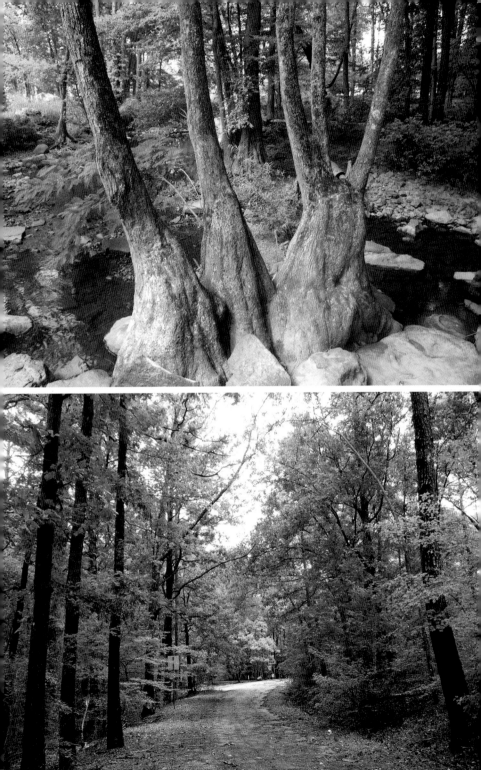

Boyle Park – East

South Nature Trail

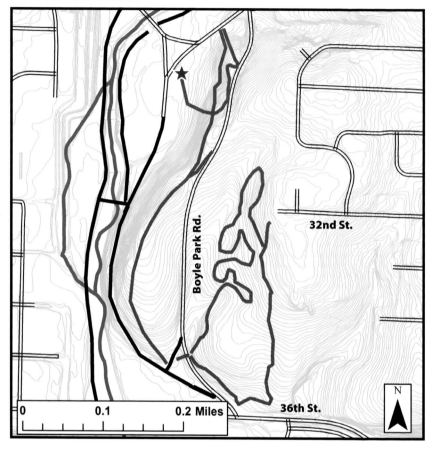

Start: 34°43' 33.8"N 92°21' 26.6"W

End: 34°43' 16.0"N 92°21' 28.2"W

Length: 0.4 miles – One-way   **Scenery:** ★★★

Difficulty: Moderate – Steep in places, some roots and rocks in trail

This trail provides a nice unpaved alternative to the old Park Road trail that it parallels. There are several entrances to this trail on the ridge between Boyle Park Road and the paved trail along Rock Creek.

This trail begins behind pavilion #2 and goes up a steep hill. The trail gains over 30 feet in elevation very quickly which makes the first part of the trail difficult, but it levels out and passes through a wooded area which offers glimpses of Rock Creek. The trail ends after a short downhill and intersects with the paved trail near Boyle Park Road.

This trail, like many in the park, is most often used (and maintained) by bikers, so be alert if you are traveling on foot!

To make this trail longer, catch the Nun Trail located across Boyle Park Rd. and described on the next page.

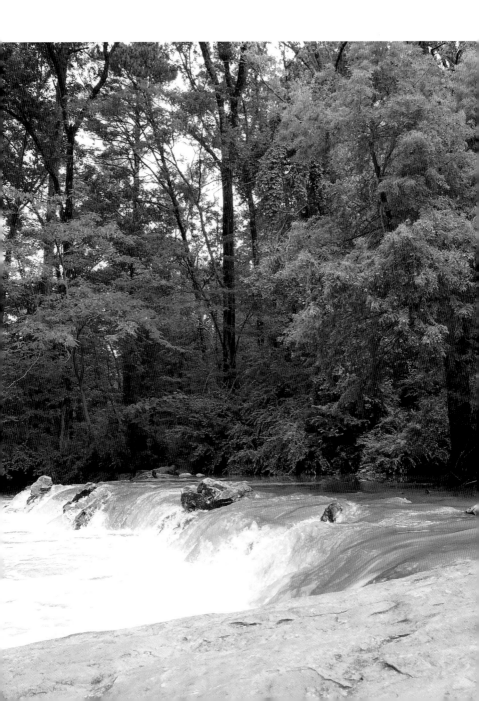

Nun Trail

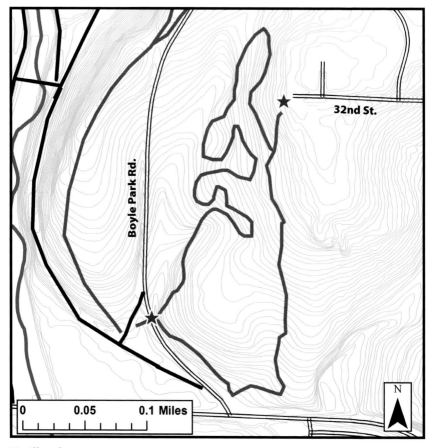

Trailheads:

Boyle Park Road: 34°43'17.14"N 92°21'26.76"W

32nd Street: 34°43'25.51"N 92°21'19.51"W

Length: 0.9 mile – Loop   **Scenery:** ★★★

Difficulty: Moderate – Moderate elevation change and rocky

With entrances at Boyle Park Road and 32nd Street, this nearly one-mile loop winds its way through a forested area in the southeastern corner of Boyle Park. Used primarily by mountain bikers, the western half of the trail has several twists and turns. The eastern half is much straighter and runs along a fence for much of its length.

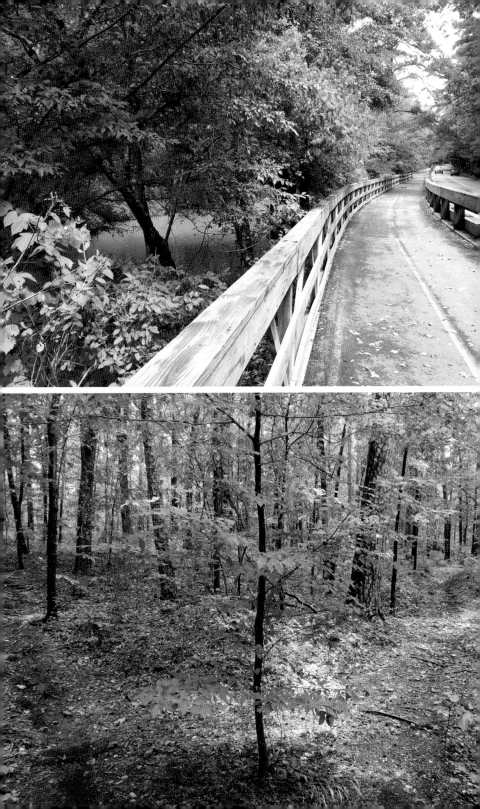

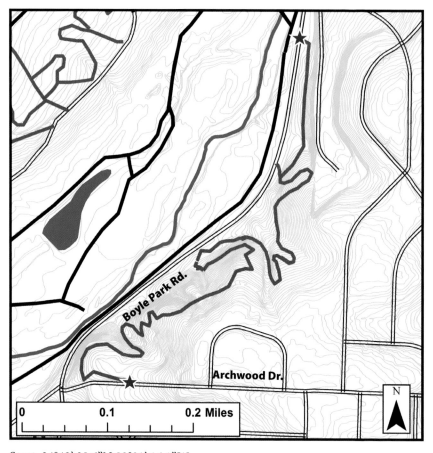

Start: 34°43' 38.6"N 92°21' 16.1"W

End: 34°43' 57.0"N 92°21' 01.8"W

Length: 0.9 miles – One-way   **Scenery:** ★★★✦

Difficulty: Hard – Lots of elevation change and rocky

The extremely winding trail twists it way through an area bounded by Boyle Park Rd., Archwood Dr., and the Broadmoor neighborhood to the east of the park. Designed by mountain bikers, this trail doesn't get you anywhere quickly, but it really crams a fairly scenic hike into a small area in the middle of Little Rock. Paralleling about half a mile of Boyle Park Rd., it covers nearly a mile. The trail starts at Archwood Dr. about 175 yards east of Boyle Park Rd., heading west and slightly downhill. This trail contains a lot of 180 degree turns and has numerous up and down hills. After about 450 yards and seven sharp turns the trail levels out for a while before beginning the twists and turns again. The final 350 yards of the trail is straight and flat and the trail ends near the Boyle Park sign with a bridge connecting paved trails on both sides of the creek.

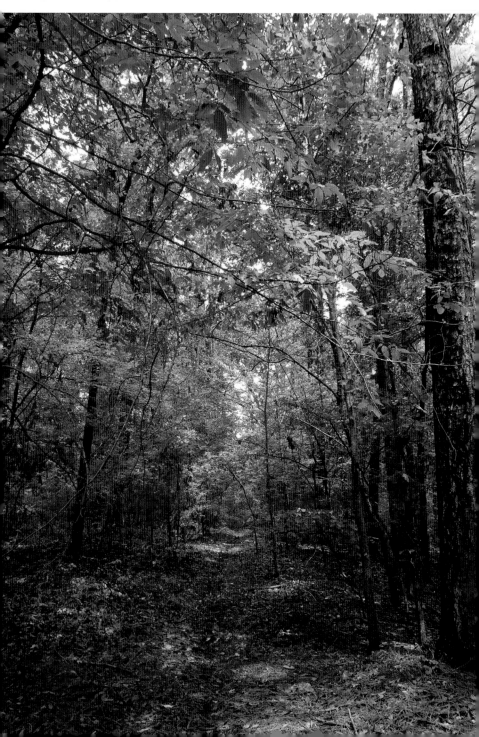

Boyle Park – West

Boyle Park West Outer Trail

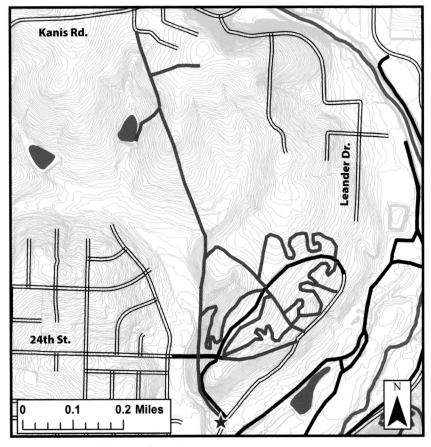

Start: 34°43'46.98"N 92°21'32.33"W

Length: 2.17 miles - Loop   **Scenery:** ★★★★

Difficulty: Moderate – Some elevation change and rocky in places

Get on the dirt trail that begins in Boyle Park near where some large boulders block off an old paved road from the main road running through the western part of the park. Follow this fairly straight trail that runs along a gas pipeline right of way for 0.8 miles. Near Kanis, short spurs lead to a small lake on one side and an apartment complex on the other. You might consider turning around at this point, since a fairly aggressive, unchained dog roams the trailer park where the trail hits Kanis. Heading back the way you came, take a left shortly after you re-cross the small stream.

Follow this trail uphill for a tenth of a mile. Shortly before it hits the paved loop, the dirt trail forks. Take a sharp left and follow the dirt trail for 0.4 miles as it winds its way though the woods. At one point you will see a barbed wire fence. Shortly before you reach the fence you may see a less worn trail head off to the left, but be sure to stay right. The trail makes several sharp turns before straightening and intersecting the paved loop.

Take a left on the paved trail and then a right when you hit the road. Follow the road for a third of a mile to get back to where you started or explore some of the numerous other trails in the vicinity.

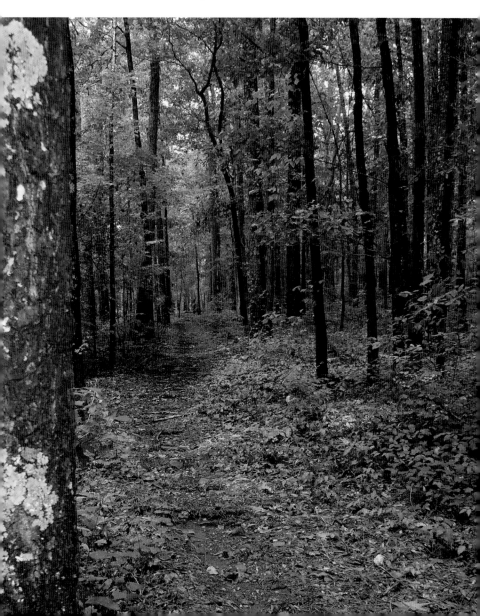

Boyle Park West Inner Loop Trail

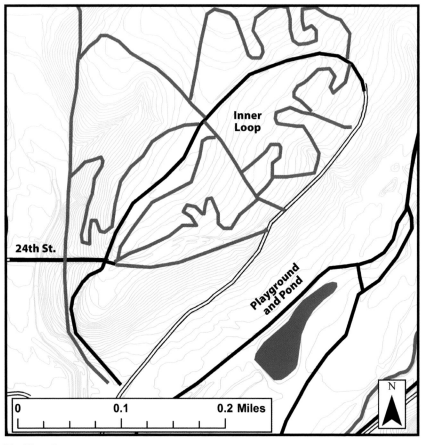

Trailheads:

1. 34°43'54.46"N 92°21'21.26"W   3. 34°43'58.63"N 92°21'26.09"W

2. 34°44'01.33"N 92°21'15.97"W   4. 34°43'52.68"N 92°21'31.54"W

Scenery: ★★★↲

Difficulty: Moderate – slightly steep, rocky in places

This trail winds it way around the interior of the paved loop that is formed by an active road and a closed-off road that is currently accessible only to bikers and pedestrians. This dirt trail can be accessed from many points around the paved loop and zig-zags around, cramming about 1,300 yards of trail into a relatively small area.

Brodie Creek

Flowing from West Little Rock southeast until it joins Fourche Creek in Hindman Park, Brodie Creek is one of the most scenic creeks in town. This hidden gem doesn't have much in the way of developed trails, but for more adventurous readers these sites will amaze you with how far from civilization they make you feel while being surrounded by the city.

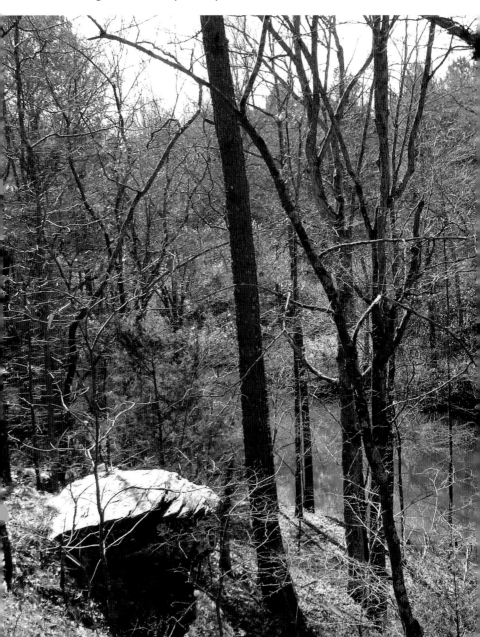

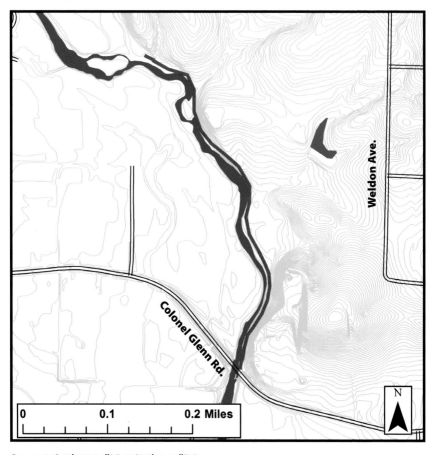

Start: 34°42' 37.94"N 92°23' 6.46"W

End: 34°42' 53.10"N 92°23' 9.45"W

Length: 0.3 miles – one-way   **Scenery:** ★★★★✦.

Difficulty: Easy – fairly flat, but rough in places

This hike is one of my favorites in Little Rock. The scenery is outstanding. Large quartz infused boulders line mossy banks where large pines grow next to cypress trees. In the spring trout lilies, rue anemone, and other interesting flowers bloom along the trail. For much of the hike you have the clear waters of Brodie Creek flowing through cypress knees on one side and a steep forested hillside with rocky outcroppings on the other.

This trail begins on the north side of the Colonel Glenn bridge over Brodie Creek, just 700 yards west of the intersection with Stagecoach Rd. Parking on the street can be a bit scary so you might try parking at AIMCO about 200 yards west of the bridge or in the nearby neighborhood.

Hiking along the right side of the creek, you will enter a beautiful forested area with a steep hillside on your right and Brodie Creek on your left. For the most part the trail is easy to follow, but in places it is overgrown. If you lose the trail your best bet is to just stay close to the creek until you find it again.

As you make your way along the creek, you'll pass several islands of varying sizes. Shortly after crossing a small ephemeral stream and passing a small island, you'll come across what is perhaps simultaneously the most scenic and unsightly part of the trail. An overturned bullet riddled car and several appliances mar a setting that you could otherwise confuse with being somewhere in Petit Jean State Park. The car lies on a steep hillside with a large rock overhang. Climbing this hill gives you a great view of the area. In the creek there is a big island lined with large river birch and pine.

A bit further up the creek you reach a point where a tributary and two branches of Brodie Creek come together. These can be hard to cross without getting wet, and just upstream the vegetation gets REALLY thick, making this a good point to turn around. If you aren't quite ready to turn around, feel free to turn to the right and explore the area around the smaller tributary.

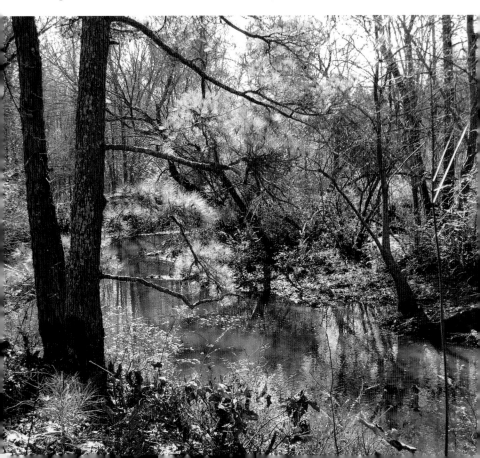

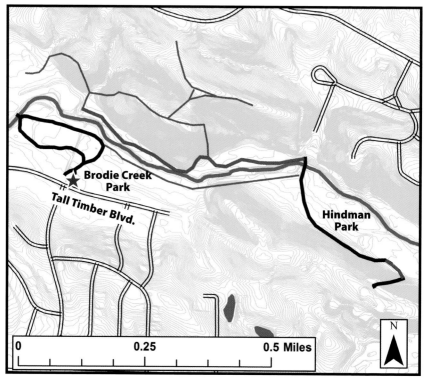

Start: 34°42'6.25"N 92°22'29.73"W

End: 34°42'4.70"N 92°22'8.17"W

Length: 0.35 miles – One-way   **Scenery:** ★★★↲

Difficulty: Moderate – trail overgrown at times, steep side trails

Another section of Brodie Creek that is particularly scenic lies between Brodie Creek Park and Hindman Park. There is a dirt trail along the north side of the creek that is easy to follow in late fall and winter, but can be overgrown by the end of summer.

I like to park at Brodie Creek Park, located on Tall Timber Blvd. about 1/3 mile east of Stagecoach Rd., between Shackleford Rd. and Colonel Glenn. From the parking lot, head north to the creek. I typically cross near the eastern edge of the grassy area and pick up the dirt trail on the other side. Head east along the trail, keeping the creek on your right. In the spring you will encounter beautiful large patches of yellow and white trout lilies growing in this forested area of cypress, tupelo, oaks, and pines. After about 600 yards, the trail reaches Hindman Golf Course. This makes a good turning around point if you are mostly interested in hiking more natural, forested locales; however the golf course can be quite scenic in its own right and is a good place to view wildlife. Great Blue Herons and beaver frequent the course's creeks and ponds, and spotted gar can be seen in Fourche Creek.

If the creek is too high to cross, you can follow the sewer right-of-way along the southern side of the creek, but this hike is much less scenic.

You can also avoid crossing Brodie Creek by hiking this route in reverse. Park at the golf club parking lot up on the hill in Hindman Park, walk out the west side of parking lot and follow the paved cart trail down hill for almost 100 yards. Turn left (north) and walk down the steep grassy hillside about 200 feet until you reach another cart trail. Turn left on the trail and follow it around the edge of the golf course for almost a third of a mile. Right after you cross Brodie Creek on the bridge, look to your left for a way into the woods. There are a few spots that all lead back to the trail, just make sure you find the trail that runs along the creek and heads west.

*The thinner trails shown on the north side of the creek are currently on private property and should be avoided. They are included here for orientation purposes.

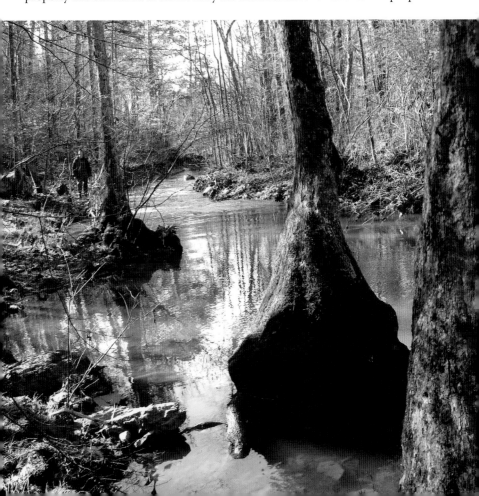

Burns Park

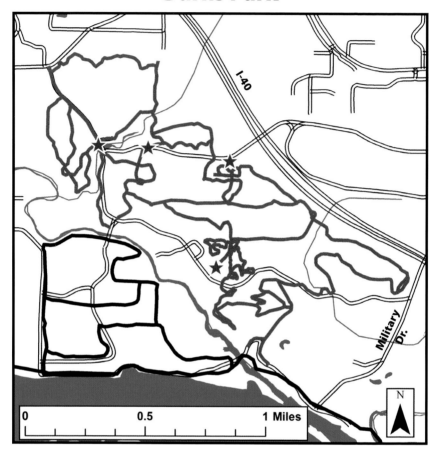

Occupying 1,700 acres in western North Little Rock, this massive park is home to baseball fields, an amusement park, a BMX course, dozens of soccer/ultimate frisbee fields, a campground, and miles and miles of paved and unpaved, bike, equestrian, and pedestrian trails.

Located at the Military Dr. exit of I-40, the park is a great place for mountain bikers, with miles of challenging trails and bike specific features like small dirt ramps and sharp, banked turns with none of the hassles of registering at nearby Camp Robinson. The Master Naturalists and the city are frequently making modifications to old trails and creating new ones, so be sure to visit the website or visitors center for up-to-date information.

Main Parking Areas (all on Burns Park Dr):

Middle, Main Access Point 34°48'9.33"N 92°19'0.16"W

BMX Course: 34°47'49.91"N 92°19'4.32"W

Covered Bridge/Yellow Trail Parking 34°48'16.31"N 92°19'30.83"W

Equestrian Trail Parking 34°48'14.49"N 92°19'23.04"W

Given the maze of overlapping trails present and the fact that multiple new trails and alternate routes for existing trails were under development at the time of this writing, I've provided basic summaries of some trails in different parts of the park, but the best approach might be to grab some water and just explore.

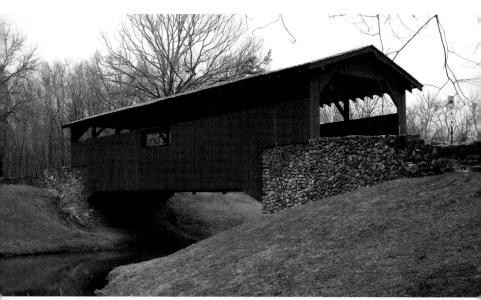

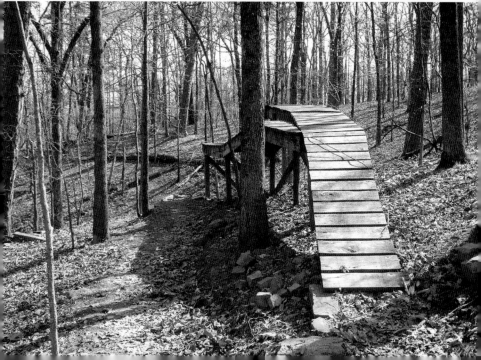

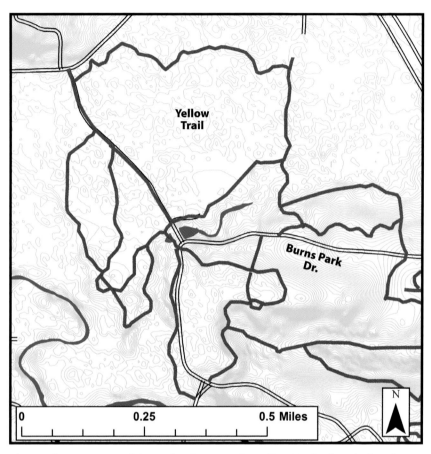

The northwest corner of the park is home to the Yellow Trail, a largely flat, dirt and gravel trail that is in relatively good shape. Though there are many interesting things to see along this trail, be sure to check out the large sycamore near the Soccer Fields.

Burns Park - Central

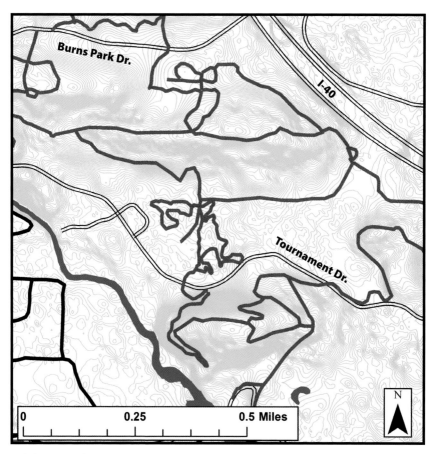

While most of the trails in the park seem popular with mountain bikers, the trails right around the BMX track were made with mountain bikers in mind. While I had fun running in tight zigzags and crazy loops over little humps and banked turns to map this area, I could see how these trails would be more fun on a bike. Directly to the south of this area, the green trail has some amazing ramps and other mountain biking features on it.

Cadron Settlement

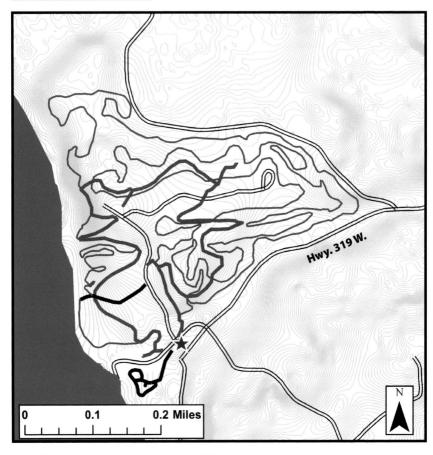

Start/End: 35° 6'16.66"N 92°32'38.07"W

Length: 1.3 miles – Loop   **Scenery:** ★★★★

Difficulty: Moderate – gravel, rocky and steep in places

Located along the Arkansas River, west of Conway off Hwy. 319, Cadron Settlement Park is home to a dense network of walking and mountain biking trails. A 4.2 mile mountain biking trail (thin red line on map) surrounds, crisscrosses, and in places overlaps a 1.3 mile (thicker red line) gravel walking trail in this mostly wooded and hilly park. There are two short, paved handicap accessible trails in the park. The northern one heads 0.1 miles west from a parking area to a spot with a nice view of the Arkansas River. The southern one takes visitors 0.2 miles past large mountains of sand at the neighboring sand company, through an open cedar grove with multiple educational signs that discuss the historic significance of the site which had a role in both the Trail of Tears and the Civil War.

The 1.3 mile gravel Tollantusky Trail begins at the main parking area near the entrance of the park. Facing north from the parking area you will see a sign and the trail heading into the woods in two places. Take the section of the trail off to the left near the spring. The trail heads slightly uphill for 0.1 miles before forking. Though faded blazes can cause some confusion, the Tollantusky Trail is marked with orange blazes while the mountain bike trail is marked with yellow. The mountain bike trail heads off to the left, while the Tollantusky Trail goes to the right. Both will take you to the same place; a lookout with a nice view of the Arkansas River. If you take the Tollantusky, you will need to turn left at the paved trail to get to the lookout.

After enjoying the view, head back the way you came on the paved trail, past the mountain bike trail, and turn left at the orange blaze. Both trails again take you to the same place, another lookout, but the mountain bike trail is twice as long and covers rougher terrain.

Following the Tollantusky, the path heads mostly uphill for the next 0.3 miles to a pavilion and another nice view of the Arkansas River. From the pavilion, the trails overlap briefly as you travel north. At the next split, be sure to take a right to stay on the Tollantusky, unless you want a much longer hike. From this point, the mountain bike trail traces the perimeter of the park and doesn't intersect the walking trail again for over a mile. Following the Tollantusky east, you will cross a different section of the mountain bike trail twice before coming to a paved road after 0.25 miles. There are picnic tables and restrooms around the parking area here.

The trail continues on the other side of the road. Soon the trail parallels the bike trail closely before crossing it. After a sharp right turn, the trail heads downhill for 0.2 miles, crossing the bike trail twice. At the next intersection, turn left and follow the combined trails 200 yards back to the parking lot.

Camp Robinson Special Use Area

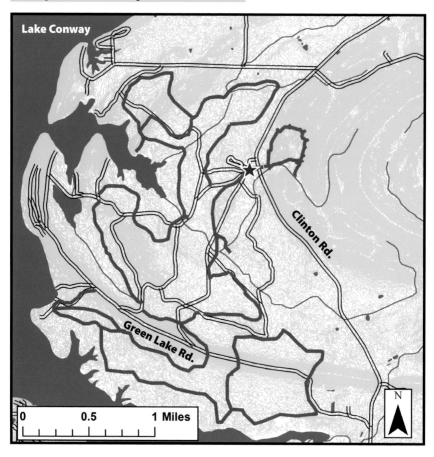

Start/End: 34°59'32.16"N 92°21'32.87"W

Scenery: ★★★★

Difficulty: Moderate – flat and long.

Camp Robinson Special Use Area is located east of Mayflower on Hwy 89, near Grassy Lake. In addition to over 15 miles of horse and hiking trails, this 4,000 acre management area has great places to fish, hunt, camp, train hunting dogs, and practice archery.

Be sure to check the website for scheduling, as hiking is not allowed when other events (there are lots of them) are taking place.

The special use area has made use of controlled burns for decades in order to maintain lots of open oak savannah and prairie habitat on the property. The diversity of habitats present including wetlands, prairies, lakes, open forest and dense pine forest make the SUA a great place for birding. In fact, the property is designated an Important Bird Area by the National Audubon Society due to sightings of Bachman's Sparrow and Bell's Vireo in addition to many species of warblers, sparrows, and shorebirds.

This area is so large and trails are poorly labeled, so the best approach here would be to just grab some water and explore. If it has rained recently, be prepared to cross lots of streams. My favorite spots include the lake and wetland areas as well as the large open grasslands since most hikes in Arkansas are through dense woods.

A good place to park and get information (marked with a star on the map) is on Nursery Pond Rd. just west of Clinton Rd.

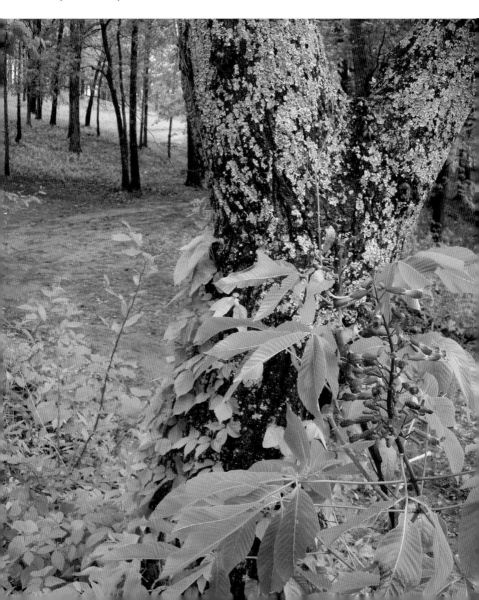

Conner Park

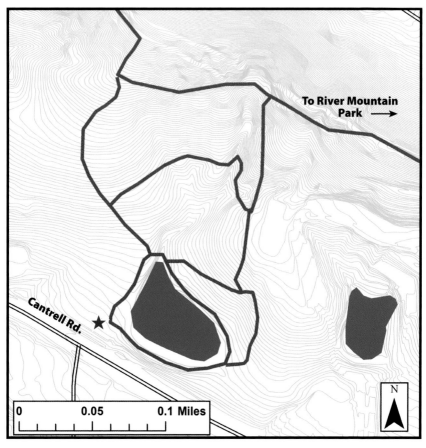

Start/End: 34°47'59.51"N 92°25'6.97"W

Length: 0.6 miles – Loop   **Scenery:** ★★★★

Difficulty: Moderate – steep in places

Located on Cantrell Rd. just west of Sam Peck Rd., Conner Park is home to four short trails and a fishing pond. The Blue Trail makes a short, easy loop around the pond, while at a little over half a mile, Yellow is the most difficult.

My favorite is taking the Yellow Trail uphill to the power line right-of-way. Turning left at the power line and heading west will earn you some great views of West Little Rock and Chenal Mountain. Taking a right at the powerline will eventually lead you to Southridge Rd. and the uphill end of the River Mountain Trail (pg. 98) which in turn connects to the River Trail (pg. 100) and Two Rivers Park (pg. 122).

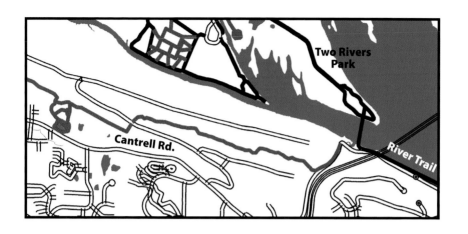

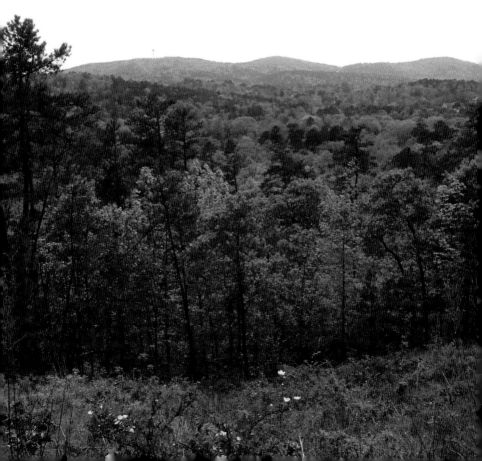

Dupree Park

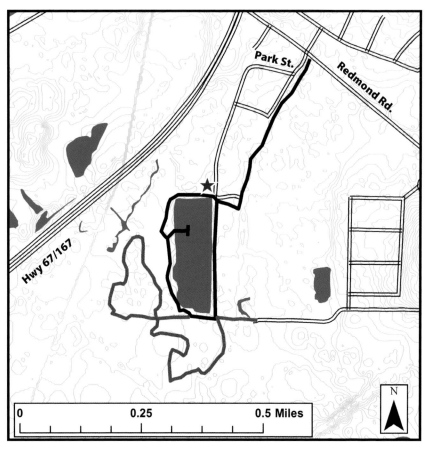

Start/End: 34°51'21.47"N 92° 7'51.99"W

Length: 1.0 mile – Loop   **Scenery:** ★★★

Difficulty: Easy – paved and flat

Dupree Park is located on Park Street off of Redmond Rd. in Jacksonville right next to Hwy 67/167. The park is home to baseball fields, soccer fields, a paved walking trail, and an 18-hole disc golf course. The 7-8' asphalt walking trail passes ball fields and runs around a lake. There are some wooden piers that provide nice places to sit and/or fish.

For a softer trail and slightly wilder experience, try walking the disc golf course that winds through the woods in the southwestern corner of the park. While dodging flying frisbees, look for large water birds along the creek and enjoy the shade of good-sized sweet gum, water oak, or cypress.

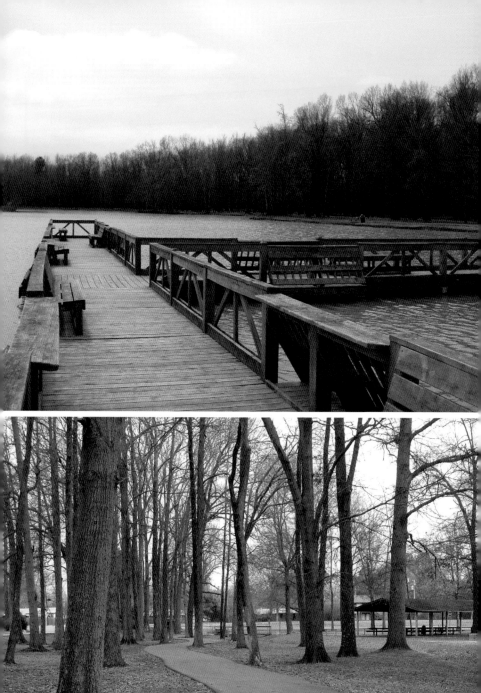

Emerald Park

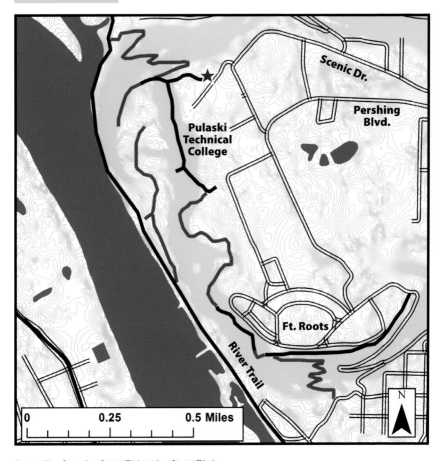

Start/End: 34°47'2.95"N 92°18'2.73"W

Length: 4.0 miles – Loop   **Scenery:** ★★★★★

Difficulty: Moderate – steep and rocky in places, paved and flat in others

Emerald Park is located near Pulaski Tech on Marge Gardner Ln. off of Scenic Drive in North Little Rock. The site of an old quarry, this park is home to dramatic red bluffs with great views of the Arkansas River and Little Rock. After heavy rains, multiple waterfalls plunge 80'–90' over the edge of the bluffs creating an extraordinary sight. This trail runs along the top of the bluff and connects to the River Trail (pg. 100) in two places; making it a great side-trip for people looking for a bit more exercise than the flat, paved, River Trail offers.

From the parking lot, follow the paved trail west. In 200 yds. the trail forks. To the right is a pavilion and access to a dirt path that heads down to the River Trail. Stay left at the fork and follow the paved trail along the top of the cliffs. There are lots of dirt side-trails throughout this section with nice views, but there is a safer, paved side-trail just 440 yards down the path and 175 yards past this lookout, the pavement ends and the trail is made of crushed asphalt and gravel.

The trail becomes rockier as it winds through a wooded area for another half mile before coming to a fence at Ft. Roots. Just past the fence, the trail is once again paved. This section of the trail is open, has great views, and several benches. The paved trail continues along the top of the cliff all the way to Ft. Roots Dr. where there is a small parking area.

To complete the loop though, turn right onto the dirt trail just past the benches and near the power line crossing. The trail heads downhill via switchbacks for the next half mile. When you reach the road, take a right on it and then another right in 175 yards to get on the River Trail near the skate park. Side trails, located half a mile or more down the River Trail offer detours up to the base of the cliffs. A half mile after the last of these detours, you should see a sign for Emerald Park pointing to a dirt trail on the right. If you cross a bridge on the River Trail, you've gone too far.

The rocky and steep trail follows switchbacks uphill for nearly half a mile before reaching the paved trail near the pavilion. Take a left and another left to get back to your car.

*The cliffs here are beautiful but dangerous. Please obey signs, stay on the trails, and keep away from the edge of the cliffs.

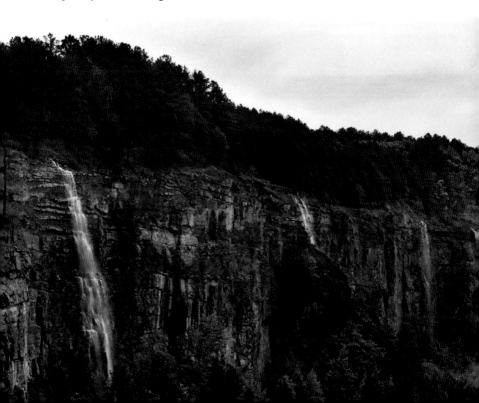

Five Mile Creek

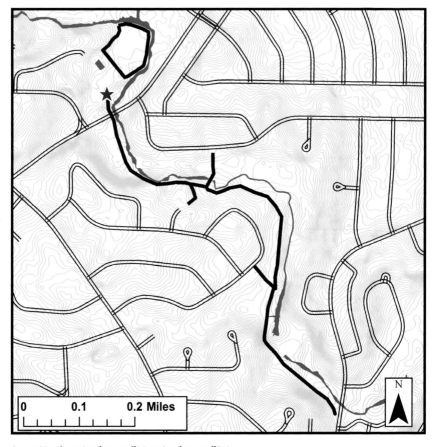

Start/End: 34°48'41.33"N 92°14'40.18"W

Length: 0.75 miles – One-way   **Scenery:** ★★★

Difficulty: Easy

This flat paved trail runs from the YMCA on JFK Blvd. to North Hills Blvd. and has several paved access points from other roads in the neighborhood. Starting at the YMCA, the asphalt trail takes you under JFK and follows Five Mile Creek for a little less than a mile. Along the way you will see scenic tupelo growing in the creek (look for wide bases and crooked trunks) and some river birch along it. Areas away from the creek are dominated by sweetgum and a mix of oaks. Perhaps the most common plant along the trail is privet, which at times forms a tunnel around the trail.

For a slightly longer walk, add the paved loop at the YMCA that winds around the softball field. More information is available online at: http://www. overbrookpoa.com/Overbrook-Trail.html.

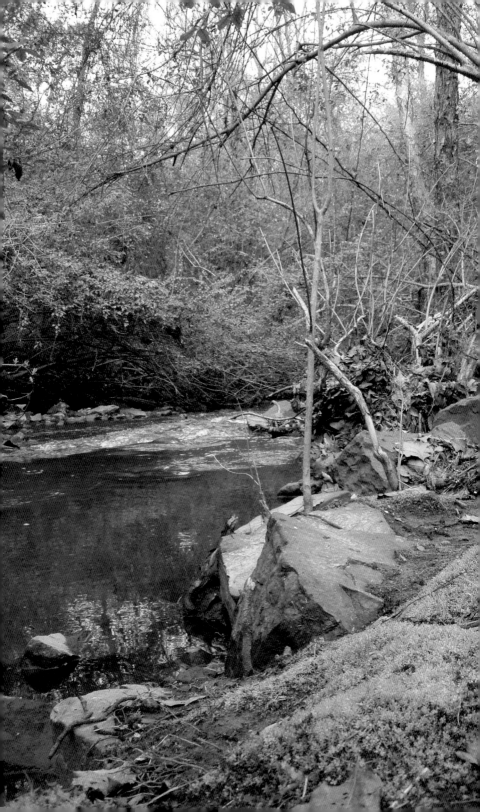

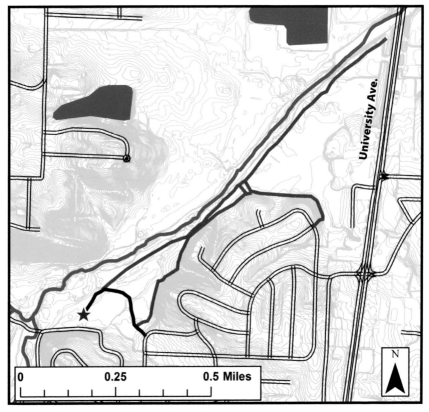

Start/End: 34°41'47.09"N 92°21'28.86"W

Length: 1.0 miles – Loop   **Scenery:** ★★★★

Difficulty: Easy – paved and flat

Hindman Park has many unique features. It is home to rare plants, a 30' out-cropping of novaculite, a canoe launch, a disc golf course, a beautiful public golf course, and miles of trails.

To get to the trail, take University Ave. to 65th St. and turn west. Follow 65th St. to the park. Once in the park, the road curves right and follows Fourche Creek. Continue along the road to where it curves right again. Park near the baseball and basketball fields and walk north to the paved trail through the open wooded area.

There are several connected trails here that take visitors along Fourche Creek, past a large rock outcropping, and through a bottomland hardwood forest.

The Meadowcliff Neighborhood Association has big plans for this park (pg. 150), including paving more of the existing trails and adding more trails to the south and north on adjacent park properties. These future trails are a part of the network of trails along Fourche Creek (pg. 149).

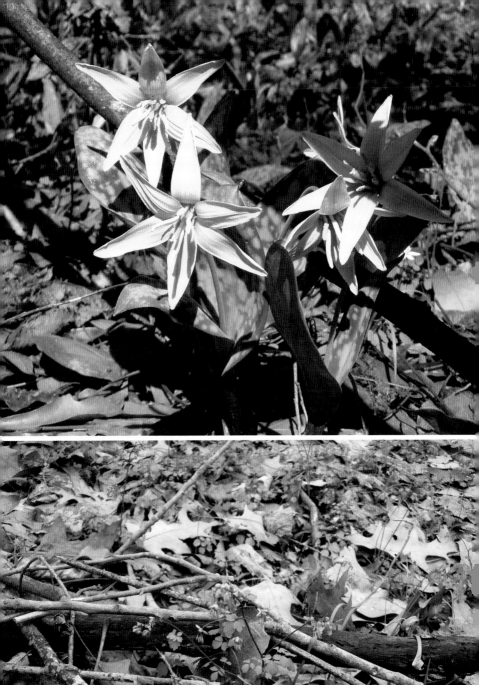
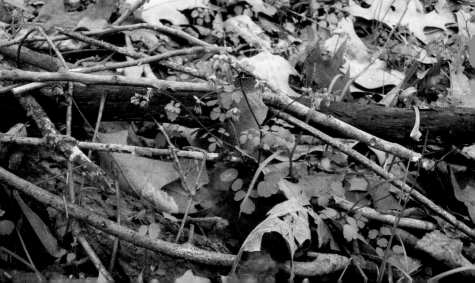

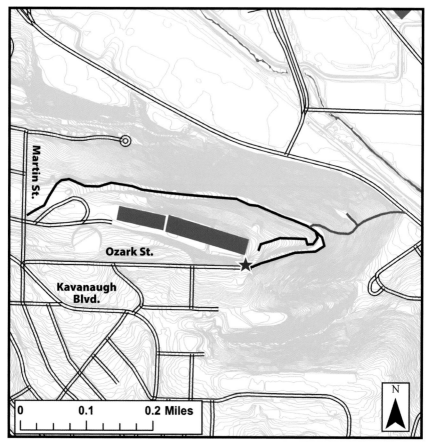

Start/End: 34°45'20.88"N 92°18'15.35"W

Length: 1.0 miles – Loop   **Scenery:** ★★★★

Difficulty: Easy – paved and flat

Knoop Park is tucked away in Hillcrest and surrounds a water treatment plant. The trail through the park is paved and fairly flat, making for a short easy walk offering stunning views of Riverdale, Downtown, and the State Capitol. If you visit the park in the spring or early summer you may catch the wisteria in bloom. To get to Knoop Park, turn north off Kavanaugh onto Fairfax Terrace and then right onto Ozark St. The road dead-ends at the entrance to Knoop Park.

From the parking area at the end of Ozark, head east along the trail until you reach the overlook area with nice benches and views of downtown Little Rock, North Little Rock, and Riverdale. This spot is a great place to watch sunrise and 4th of July fireworks. A spur trail heads off to the left up the hill and provides more views of downtown and the State Capitol.

From here the main trail heads west for about half a mile through a wooded area that is home to the large patches of wisteria mentioned above. The trail has several benches and a water fountain and ends at Martin Street. At this point you could head back the way you came or do what I like to do and make it a loop by turning left on Martin and then left on Ozark. There are some unique houses along the way featuring interesting landscaping and architectural styles.

At the north end of the lookout area with all the benches, a slightly overgrown trail heads down the hill and hits Cantrell near the River Trail. After seeing a few campfire circles and lots of trash, I'm not sure this trail is recommended.

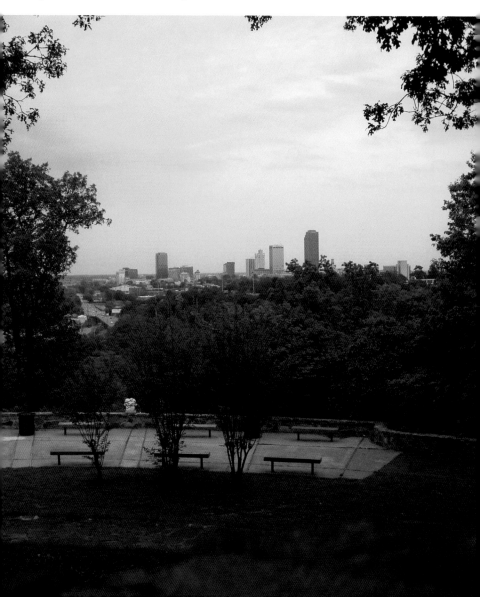

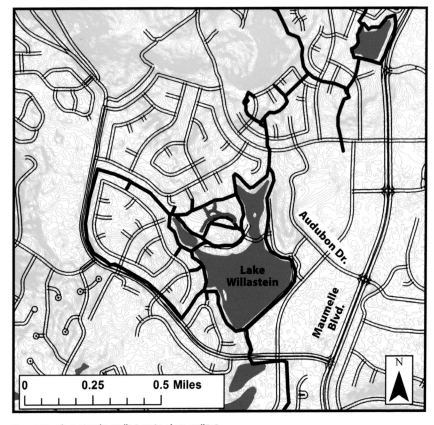

Start/End: 34°51'7.78"N 92°24'48.69"W

Length: 2.1 miles – Loop   **Scenery:** ★★★★

Difficulty: Easy – paved and flat

The City of Maumelle has an incredible network of trails connecting many parts of the city. These trails are not just glorified sidewalks, as they go many places roads don't. If you take the time to explore this maze of trails, you will come across many interesting sculptures, tunnels, small playgrounds, and bridges. The centerpiece of this vast network of trails is Lake Willastein Park, which is home to a large lake, playground, numerous picnic tables, several fishing piers, large wooden pedestrian bridges, and old bunkers that kids can explore. The roughly three miles of trail in the park form four connected loops, allowing visitors to create short or long walks through open or wooded areas. Look for parking off Lake Willastein Dr. near the intersection of Maumelle Blvd. and Odom Blvd. S.

The loop around the outer edge of the entire lake is approximately two miles. The vast majority of trails in the park are asphalt and roughly seven feet wide, however there is a short unpaved trail in the northern part of park.

Scenic Lake Valenica can be reached by trail and is about 1200 yards to the northeast of Lake Willastein Park.

For a real workout, explore the steep sections of trail around Hightrail Dr. and Millwood Circle.

Hopefully, the rapid expansion of neighboring North Little Rock won't prevent this network of trails from connecting to the River Trail in a safer manner than the current bike lane along busy Maumelle Blvd.

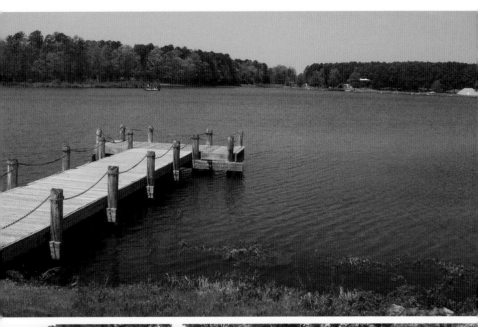

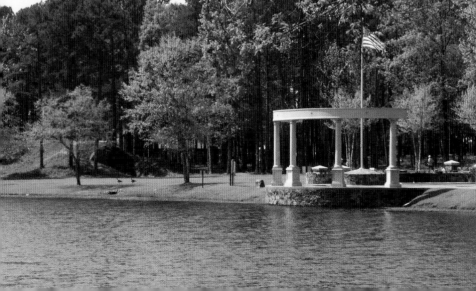

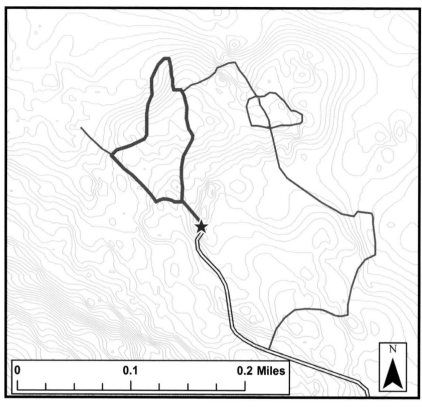

Start/End: 35° 0'8.11"N 92° 0'55.48"W

Length: 0.3 miles – Loop   **Scenery:** ★★★

Difficulty: Moderate – some elevation change, difficult to follow

Located in Cabot, off of N. Willie Ray Dr., Lonoke County Regional Park has a large BMX course, a walking trail, and lots of space for planned mountain biking trails. To get there, take Hwy 67/167 to the Main St./Hwy 89 exit in Cabot. Go west on 89 and then turn right onto Willie Ray Dr. which parallels the highway on the north side. After about two miles, turn left onto the old Willie Ray Dr. The park will be on your right before the road transitions to gravel near a watertower. Follow signs for the walking trail and park near the BMX track. The trail begins near the firing range and heads west into the woods. After ~150 yards, the trail turns sharply to the right. After another 200 yards, the trail turns to the right again and heads uphill. At this point I had a hard time following the trail. Pink and orange flagging appeared to mark a much longer trail (shown in thinner red on the map) that was slightly overgrown. If you aren't up for a little adventure, continue south to the clearing and back to your car.

*This park sometimes has odd hours. All day Saturday, and early evenings on Monday and Tuesday are good bets. Hopefully with more trails and increased use, the park will expand its open hours.

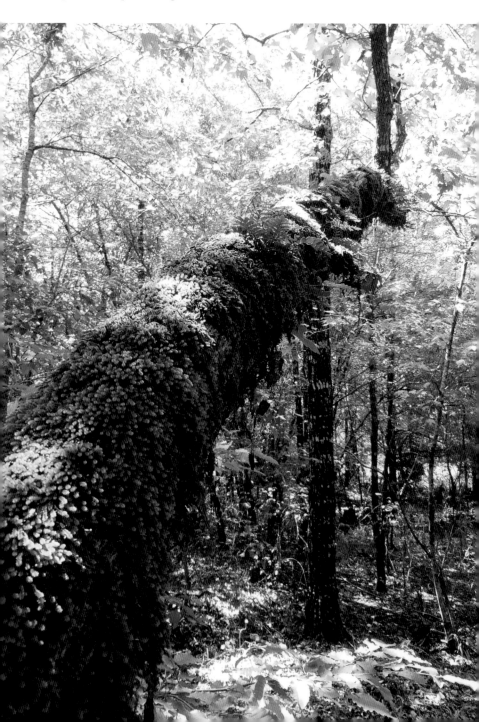

Lorance Creek Natural Area

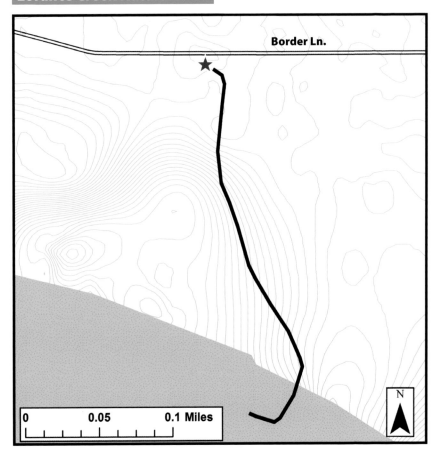

Start/End: 34°35'12.89"N 92°15'14.03"W

Length: 0.5 miles – In and Out   **Scenery:** ★★★✦.

Difficulty: Easy – paved and flat

Lorance Creek Natural Area is located 10 miles south of Little Rock, on Border Ln., a mile east of the Bingham Rd. exit off of I-530. Starting from the parking area, the 6 foot asphalt-like, "resin pave" trail heads south through an upland pine/oak forest. There are numerous educational signs along the way describing the history and ecological significance of the site. After 350 yards, the trail transitions to a boardwalk and continues through a scenic cypress/tupelo swamp. Along the roughly 400 feet of boardwalk, look for woodpeckers and warblers, while listening for the bird-voiced treefrog.

More information on the natural area can be found at:
http://www.naturalheritage.com/natural-area/lorance-creek/

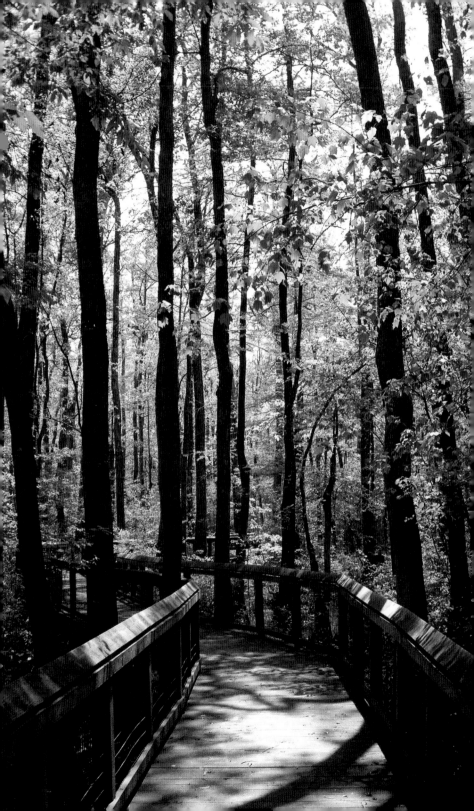

Maumelle River WMA

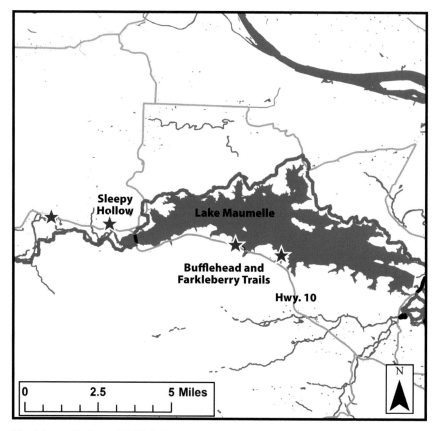

The Maumelle River Wildlife Management Area is a new WMA that surrounds Lake Maumelle and a good chunk of the Maumelle River upstream of the lake. The WMA allows floating and some hunting in certain areas. Sleepy Hollow Park on Hwy. 10 has a nice boat launch and another launch will likely be built a few miles upstream of there. The Maumelle River is quite scenic and less busy than the nearby Little Maumelle.

In addition to the lengthy Ouachita Trail, which travels the entire north side of the lake, there are two short trails on the south side that offer views of the lake. Of the two, I prefer the Bufflehead Trail, which is slightly longer than its neighbor to the west, the Farkleberry Trail. It doesn't hurt that I saw a spotted gar swimming near the trail while walking the Bufflehead. If trying to decide between the two trails, just pick whichever one you enjoy saying more.

More information and a map can be found at the following links:

http://www.agfc.com

http://www.agfc.com/resources/maps/Maumelle%20River.pdf

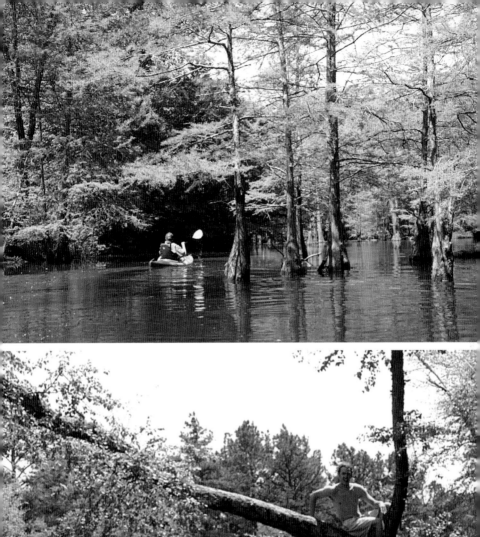
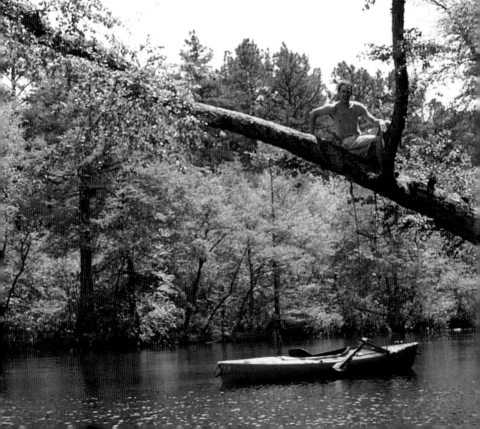

Mills Park

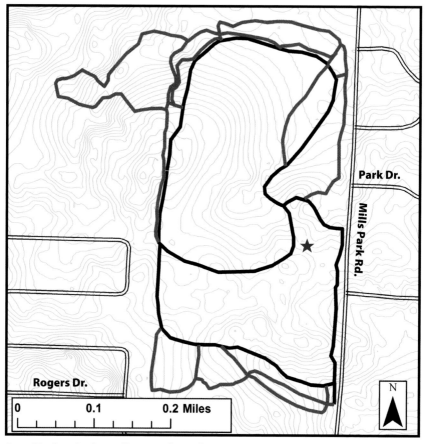

Start/End: 34°36'18.71"N 92°28'57.12"W

Length: 1.3 miles – Loop   **Scenery:** ★★★✦

Difficulty: Easy – paved and flat

Located along Mills Park Rd. just over a mile south of I-30, Mills Park is a Bryant City Park that is partially managed by the Arkansas Natural Heritage Commission due to the presence of rare plants and a unique acid seep ecosystem.

The park features two overlapping paved loops, one mostly forested, the other mostly open. Unpaved trails ring the paved loops, and take visitors to less busy parts of the park.

A trip around the outer paved loop covers a little more than one mile. In early to mid- April, the woods inside the loop are full of dogwoods in bloom. Slightly earlier in the spring, you may see a good number of redbuds as well. The woods at the northern part of the loop contain dense stands of pine, though this is likely to change gradually as intentional thinning and controlled burns continue to take place.

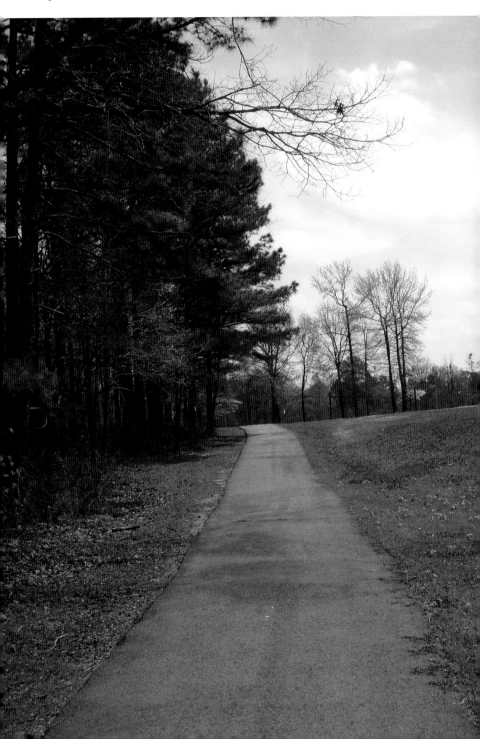

Ouachita Trail

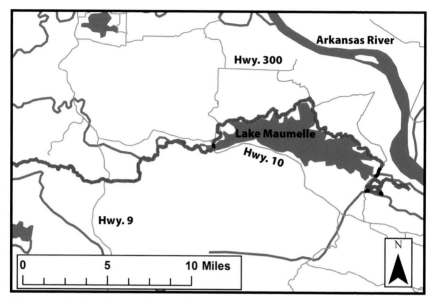

The 223 mile Ouachita Trail runs from Pinnacle Mountain State Park to Talimena State Park in Oklahoma. In Central Arkansas, it heads west from the park visitor center, around the north side of Lake Maumelle, along the Maumelle River, through some forested hills, and passes near Lake Sylvia before continuing west through the Ouachita National Forest. The stretch between Hwy. 10 and Hwy. 9 is much more scenic than the section around Lake Maumelle where views of the lake are few and far between. The trail is marked with blue blazes and white diamond mile-markers. Make sure you keep your eye out for these, as the trail crosses and overlaps many old roads, utility right-of-ways, and other trails. I lost the trail multiple times when hiking it in August, so for that and many other reasons, fall and winter are the best times to do this trail.

Main Access Locations:

Pinnacle Mountain Visitor Center - 34°50'40.57"N 92°27'49.20"W

Spillway Rd. - 34°51'46.00"N 92°28'50.49"W

Hwy. 300 - 34°54'27.13"N 92°33'0.56"W

Hwy. 113 - 34°53'10.41"N 92°38'56.84"W

Hwy. 10 - 34°52'21.44"N 92°39'10.37"W

Hwy. 9 - 34°50'47.77"N 92°45'53.19"W

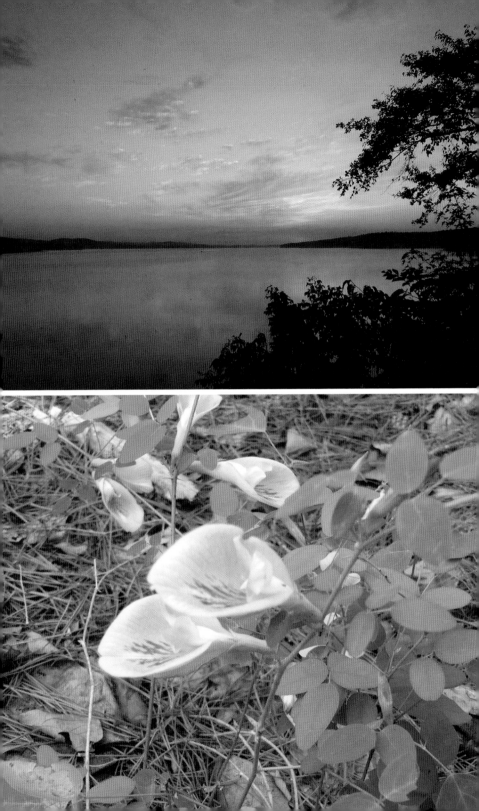

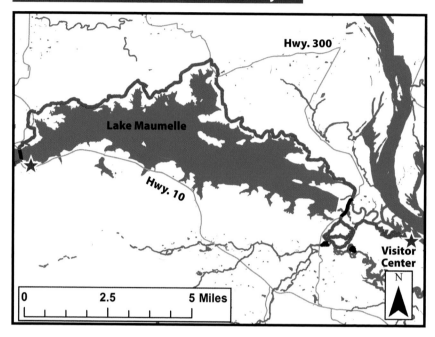

Start: 34°50'40.57"N 92°27'49.20"W

End: 34°52'21.44"N 92°39'10.37"W

Length: 21 miles – One-way   **Scenery:** ★★★✦

Difficulty: Hard – rocky in places and long

The eastern end of the Ouachita trail runs west from the Pinnacle Mountain State Park Visitor Center, around the base of Pinnacle Mountain, and then roughly parallels the shoreline of Lake Maumelle at just enough of a distance that views of the lake are uncommon. The area around the lake is full of intersecting old roads and trails, so be sure to keep an eye on the blue blazes.

The visitor center is on Pinnacle Mountain State Park Rd. about a half mile north of Pinnacle Valley Rd. You can get there from Hwy. 10 by taking Hwy. 300 or Pinnacle Valley Rd. towards the park. The trailhead is located at the far west end of the visitor center parking area.

The trail heads downhill and crosses a road to a boat launch. After nearly a mile you will cross a powerline right-of-way and then a railroad track before crossing Pinnacle Valley Rd. near the East Summit Trailhead (pg. 84). From here, the trail heads west, overlapping the Base Trail (pg. 88) for about a half mile before forking off to the right.

The trail then crosses Pinnacle Valley Rd. again. Follow Hwy. 300 north and then veer slightly to the right and take the old road. While walking across the old bridge, take in the view of a branch of the Maumelle River. In another half mile the trail crosses the spillway channel and then turns left into the woods leaving the road behind. The trail follows the spillway channel for about half a mile before reaching the Spillway Road trail access. If you've done lots of hikes at Pinnacle Mountain, this is a good place to start your hike as it cuts off a few miles and eliminates the long walk on asphalt.

As you approach the actual spillway structure, the trail turns right and heads uphill into the woods. Over the next two and a half miles the trail crosses multiple other trails and dirt roads. Many of these lead to better views of the lake, but again to stay on the Oauchita Trail, watch for those blue blazes. At this point the trail is close enough to the lake to offer views even in the middle of summer. Given the presence of ticks and view-blocking greenery, perhaps the only plus side to hiking this trail in late August is the ripe muscadines that dot the trail.

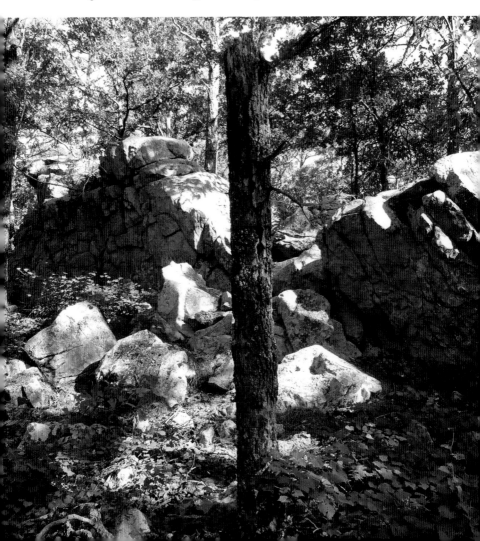

In another mile and a half you will come to a scenic lookout that offers a nice view of the lake. From here the trail shrinks a bit and heads downhill. Over the next mile and a half the trail crosses numerous small, usually dry, creek beds before straightening out and following along an old rail or road bed for a short distance. Follow the trail north for another mile and a half to reach Hwy. 300, a popular road for bicyclists. If you left a car here, the parking area is roughly 50 yards to the east.

The trail in this section is flat and soft, which is a nice change from the earlier, steeper rocky parts. Over the next 0.6 mi. the dirt and pine needle padded trail passes a small pond, crosses a gas pipeline right-of-way, and crosses Hwy. 300 again. Once again, the trail follows an old road or rail bed and is fairly straight and flat for the next 1,400 yards.

Shortly after crossing the gas pipeline right-of-way once more, the trail crosses another trail and then two large rocky ephemeral streams.

Dotted with bright purple beautyberry shrubs and butterfly pea plants in late summer, the next two miles provide additional views of the lake before arriving at the turnoff for the Penny Campsite.

Stay on the main trail. Over the next 500 yards there are two stream crossings, including one with a cable to help out during high water. After that the trail follows an old road for a short distance and then turns left.

Follow the trail a mile and a half across two more small streams and past a massive pile of sawdust to one of the best views of the lake this trail offers. The next two miles take you past two ponds, across an old road, and past a home off the right before reaching Hwy. 113. If you are tired at this point you might consider just turning left and heading south on the road, because after the trail crosses the highway, it heads briefly downhill over some rough terrain, past a pond, and then heads up a steep hill, gaining nearly 100 feet in elevation over the next 0.25 mi. From the top of the hill, it is a short walk down to Hwy. 113 and another parking area. If you parked on Hwy. 10, cross Hwy. 113 and follow the trail between the lake and the road for one mile to Hwy. 10 and cross the bridge. Be sure to take in the unimpeded views of the lake before reaching the parking area on your left.

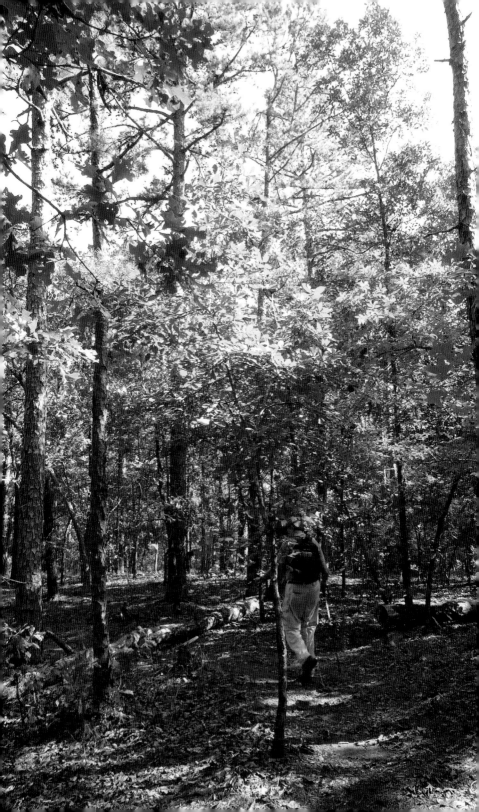

Ouachita Trail – Hwy 10 to Hwy 9

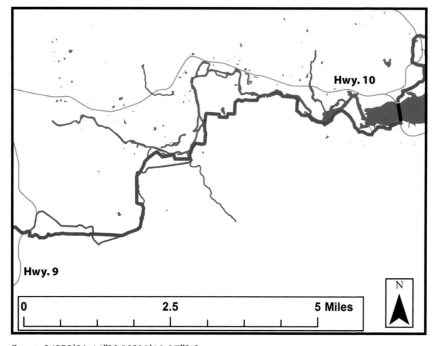

Hwy. 10

Hwy. 9

| 0 | 2.5 | 5 Miles |

N

Start: 34°52'21.44"N 92°39'10.37"W

End: 34°50'47.77"N 92°45'53.19"W

Length: 10.0 miles – One-way　　**Scenery:** ★★★★

Difficulty: Hard – long, steep in places

This section of the trail begins across Hwy. 10 from Vista Park, located at the western end of Lake Maumelle on the south side of the bridge. It is shorter and more scenic than the section discussed on the previous pages, but can be difficult to follow.

From your car, cross the road and head up the steep ladder-like steps. From here the soft, dirt and pine needle trail heads west along the Maumelle River near where it enters Lake Maumelle. Over the next mile and a half the trail meets up with a gravel road, leaves that gravel road, crosses a power line right-of-way and then meets up with the Maumelle River once again.

Follow the trail west, keeping the cypress-lined river on your right. There are three stream bed crossings in the next mile and if you lose the blue blazes, just keep the creek to your right until you find it again. In 440 yards you will pass a USGS monitoring station with a cable hung across the river. After that, the trail crosses a dirt road and continues along the river bank. Look for turkeys, mile-marker 199, and some large cypress in this area.

Approximately a half mile past the mile-marker, the trail turns sharply left and heads uphill away from the creek. Most of the trail from here on runs through or along private property. Over the next 0.6 mi. the trail is steep in places and runs along the edge of a recently logged area. You will make two sharp turns before coming to the top of a hill with an interesting rock outcropping. After you catch your breath, head down the steep hill to the high-voltage power line crossing. In summer this part can be difficult to follow and the high vegetation provides great habitat for ticks and chiggers. The trail goes straight across the first half of the right-of-way, turns right for a few yards and then heads into the woods on the other side.

From here the trail heads uphill for about 650 yards before coming to a hilltop with nice views. The next mile is hilly and provides some more views of the Maumelle River before reaching a nice gravel road and lowwater bridge. This section of the trail has changed some in the past and can be confusing. At the road, turn right and cross the bridge. The next mile runs through a hunt club property and has a couple bridges in poor condition, so you might consider just walking west down the road (shown in thin red on the map) until it meets up with the trail once again near a pipeline crossing.

The trail overlaps the road for 100 yards before heading off into the woods to the left. Head due south for half a mile and then make a couple sharp turns until you arrive at the pipeline right-of-way and a small creek. Turn right and look for the blue blazes. Follow the right-of-way south and west, across two small streams for a little over a half mile. Pay special attention to the blue blazes in this area so you don't miss where the trail departs from the right-of-way. If you happen to lose the trail in here (like I did) you can just follow the right-of-way to the road and follow it north and west to scenic Co. Rd. 153 and out to Hwy. 9 a bit north of the trailhead and parking area (this route is shown in thin red on the map).

If you are awesome and don't lose the trail, follow it almost due west for nearly two miles as it gains hundreds of feet in elevation before decending rapidly to Hwy. 9.

From here it is just 5 more miles to Lake Sylvia, which is a great place to swim, camp, hike, have a family picnic, or do an easy paddle.

Pinnacle Mountain

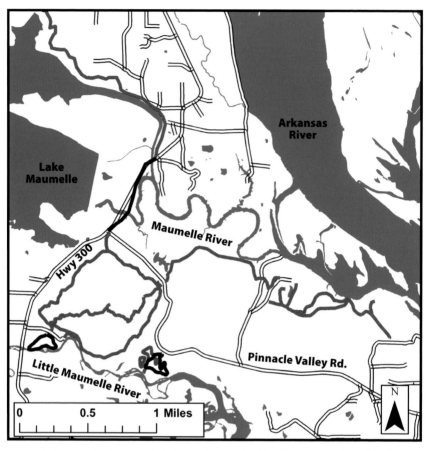

Pinnacle Mountain State Park is located near the Northwestern edge of Little Rock. The 70+ acre park has something for everyone: large fields, a playground, short paved trails through scenic bottomland forest, an arboretum, an educational visitor center, multiple put-ins on the Little Maumelle and Maumelle rivers, and several more rigorous hikes to the top of Pinnacle Mountain and other peaks in the area. The park maintains over 40 miles of paved, unpaved, and water trails. When you get to the park be sure to grab a copy of their trails brochure.

Since trails here are heavily trafficked, please stay on marked trails. Erosion is a major problem on the unpaved trails around the park and taking shortcuts or using old trails can make the problem worse.

More information on the park can be found at:
http://www.arkansasstateparks.com/pinnaclemountain/

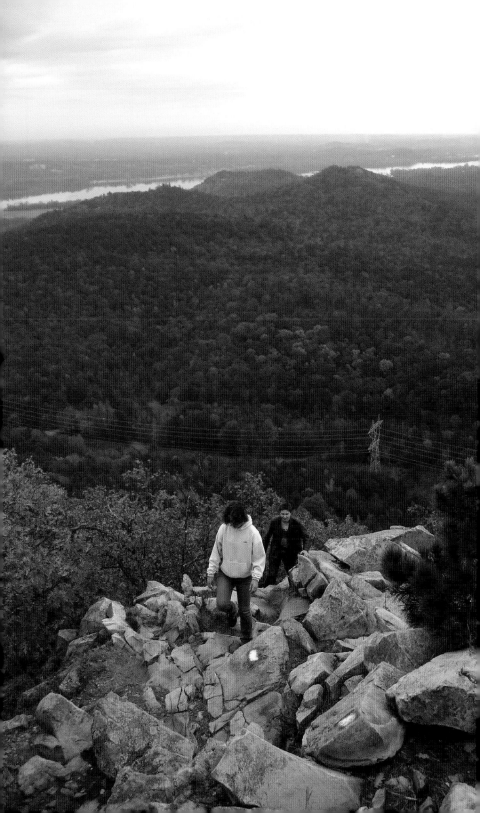

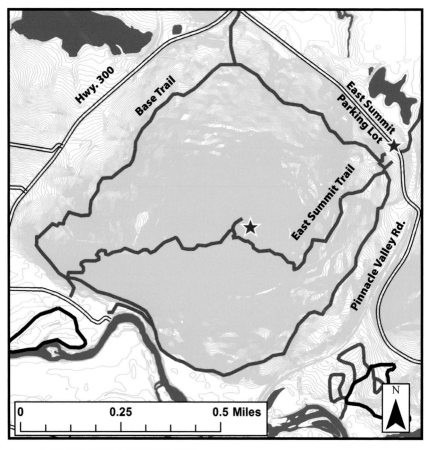

Start: 34°50'39.35"N 92°28'44.76"W

End: 34°50'29.12"N 92°29'9.13"W

Length: 0.75 miles – one-way   **Scenery:** ★★★★★

Difficulty: Very Hard – requires scrambling up steep boulder fields

This trail is the more difficult of the two trails leading to the top of Pinnacle Mountain and is perhaps the most rigorous trail in Little Rock. Parking for this trail is a half a mile east of Hwy. 300 on Pinnacle Valley Rd. Following the red and white blazes from the parking lot, the trail is initially lightly sloped and well worn. Both the East Summit and West Summit trails have markers numbered 1-10 to give you an idea of how far along the trail you are. The first six markers are deceptively easy to get to.

After that point the trail becomes very steep and involves scrambling over large boulders. Watch where you put your feet since some rocks are slick and leaf covered gaps between boulders can hide ankle twisting holes!

Since you will likely be stopping several times between markers 7 and 10, be sure to check out the amazing views along the way! If you have energy to burn, there are a of couple large rock walls around markers 8 and 9 that are fun to climb on. The trail ends at what I'll call "Peak One" which offers good views of the Arkansas River, downtown Little Rock, and Chenal Mountain to the north, east, and south. A short rocky hike to the other peak gives you great views of Lake Maumelle off to the west as well. From the top you have the option of returning the way you came or going down the easier side and walking around the base of the mountain back to your car.

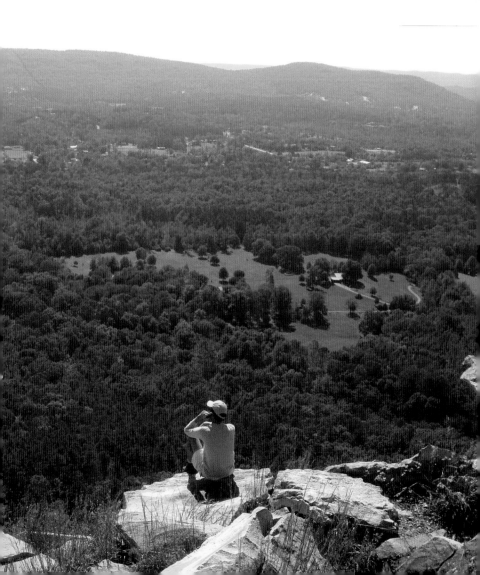

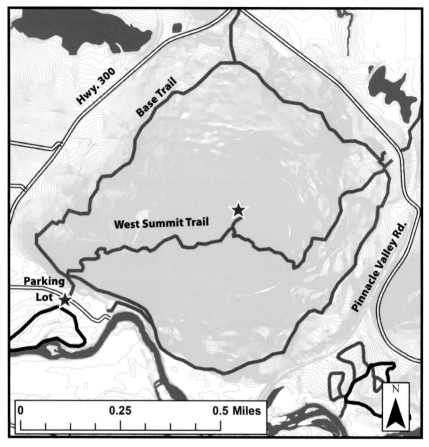

Start: 34°50'22.26"N 92°29'34.64"W

End: 34°50'31.63"N 92°29'7.62"W

Length: 0.78 miles – one-way   **Scenery:** ★★★★★

Difficulty: Hard

This is the easier of the two trails to the summit and by far the most popular. On a typical nice weekend the parking lot overflows and it isn't uncommon to pass dozens of people on your way to the top. If you prefer solitude try the East Summit Trail, explore the other summits in the park, or go when it is really cold. I've gone up this side twice without encountering a single human being; once to see sunrise on New Year's Day and the other immediately after a big ice storm.

This is a great trail to bring along the kids or dog.

The trail begins on the north side of the parking lot near the playground and restrooms. The well-worn and clearly marked trail heads gradually uphill for about 100 yards before you reach the intersection with the loop trail. Stay straight and follow signs for the West Summit Trail. About 200 yards later you will come to a short natural rock wall on your left. After almost half a mile, you will reach a large rock 'glacier' signaling that much of the rest of the trip to the top will involve hiking up large boulders. The trail is also much steeper from this point on up; luckily there are many great places to rest and take in some amazing views. As you near the top, the trail splits leading to the two different peaks. While both peaks provide near-360 degree views, the peak to the left offers better views to the north. The peak to the right has slightly better views of Little Rock and is where the East Summit trail ends.

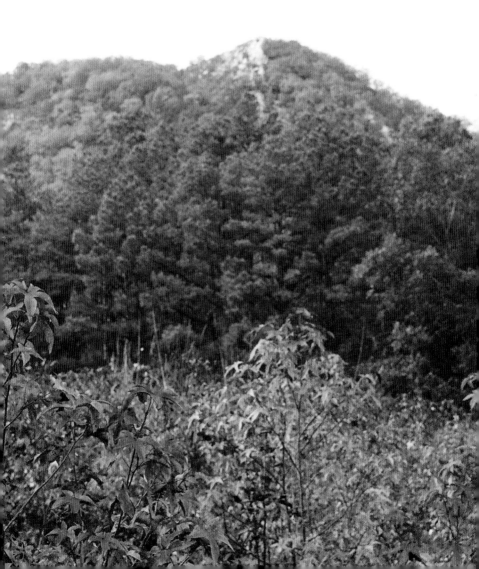

Base Trail

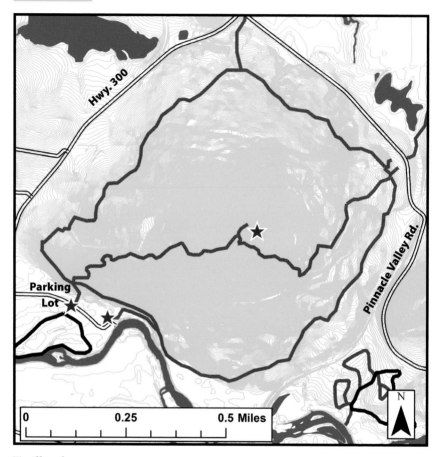

Trailheads:

West Summit Trail: 34°50'22.26"N 92°29'34.64"W

East Summit Trail: 34°50'39.35"N 92°28'44.76"W

West Side Canoe Launch: 34°50'19.80"N 92°29'28.64"W

Length: 3.0 miles – loop   **Scenery:** ★★★

Difficulty: Moderate

This trail connects the bases of the two summit trails making it possible to go up one side, down the other, and return to your car by walking around the base of the mountain. I enjoy going up the east side for more scrambling and fewer people and then down the west which is easier on the knees.

The Base Trail used to just run around the south side of the mountain, but a recently completed route around the northern side makes it possible to hike all the way around the mountain. Both sections are fairly scenic: the northern one winds through some rocky areas and past an old house while the southern route runs near the Little Maumelle for some distance. The northern route is the longer and more difficult of the two with a bit more elevation change, a rockier trail, and more switchbacks.

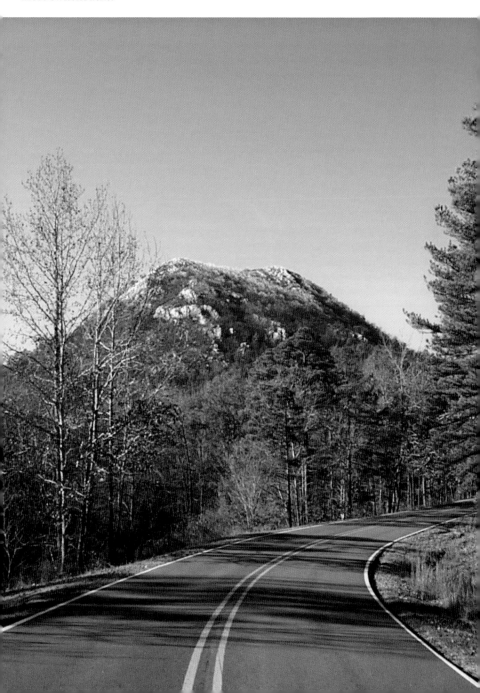

Kingfisher Trail

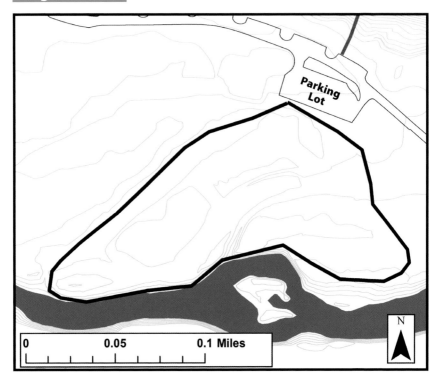

Start: 34°50'20.61"N 92°29'36.91"W

Length: 0.5 mi. - Loop   **Scenery:** ★★★★

Difficulty: Easy – short, flat, paved

The Kingfisher, perhaps the least difficult of the trails in the park, is a half mile of flat, handicapped accessible paved trail with great views of the Little Maumelle. While the trails over and around the mountain are lined with hickories, oaks, and pines; this trail is home to sycamores, river birch, sweet gums, box elders, river cane, and enormous cypress trees. A huge hollowed out cypress tree with a face-sized hole in the trunk provides a great photo op for anyone who can squeeze into the opening in the back of the tree.

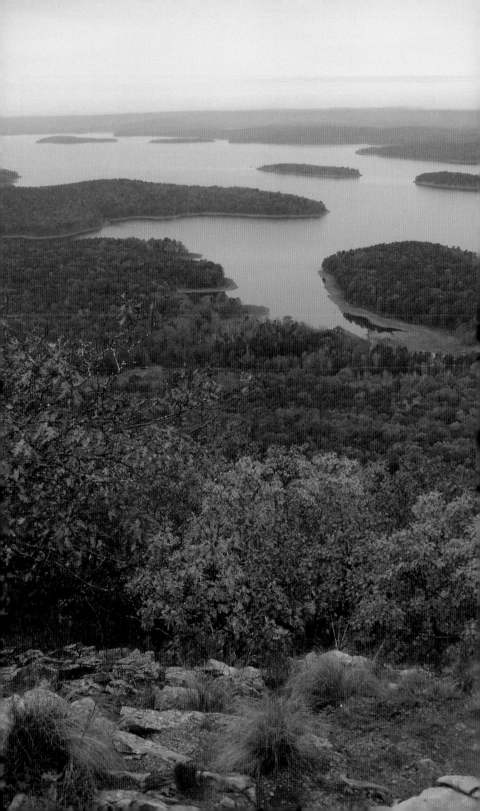

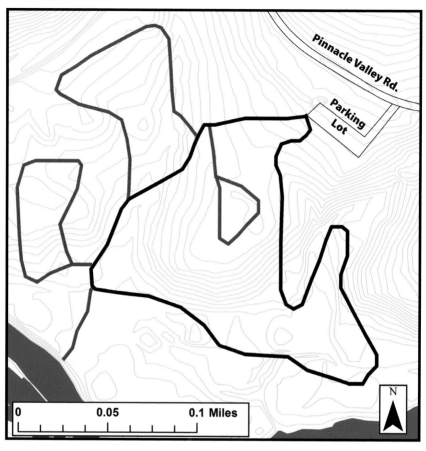

Start: 34°50'12.90"N 92°28'43.91"W

Length: 0.6 mi. - Loop   **Scenery:** ★★★↙

Difficulty: Easy – short, fairly flat, paved

The arboretum trail system consists of about a half mile of paved loop with several short dirt loop and spur trails connected to it. These trails are all fairly flat and there are plenty of benches along the way. Numerous informative signs line the trail providing information on our state's ecoregions and the species of trees found in each. Heading counter-clockwise around the trail, the fifth spur you reach will take you to a bench overlooking the Little Maumelle River.

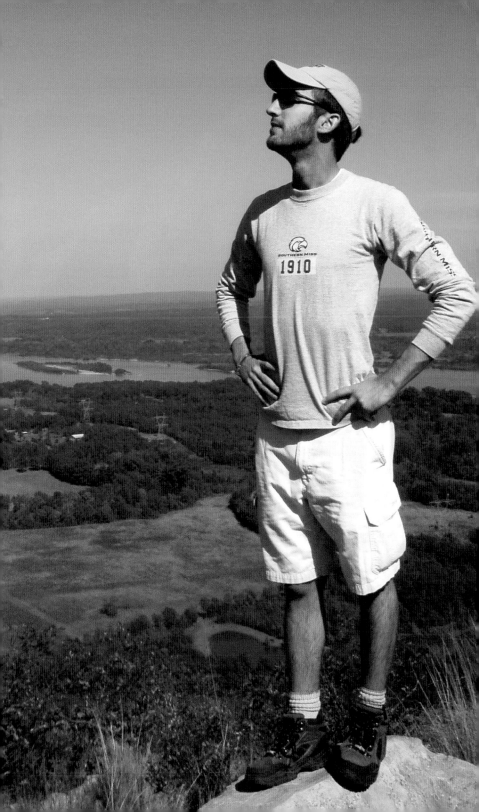

Quarry Trail

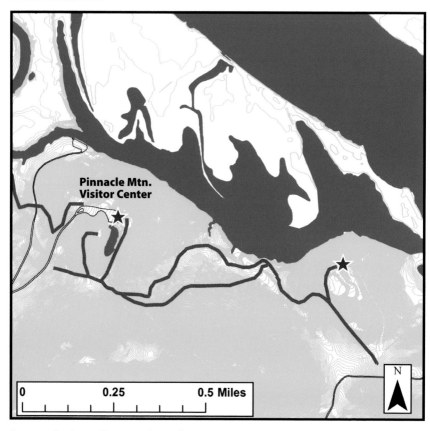

Start: 34°50'38.39"N 92°27'43.32"W

Length: 2.5 mi. - Round-Trip   **Scenery:** ★★★★

Difficulty: Moderate – steep and rocky in places

The trail begins at the southeast corner of the Pinnacle Mountain Visitor Center parking lot near the quarry pond. The trail is paved for a short while before it turns left to an overlook over the Arkansas River. To follow the quarry trail, turn right onto the dirt trail. After about 350 yards the quarry trail turns to the left. Staying straight on the road and then curving right up the hill will take you to an overlook of the quarry pond and the visitor center area.

After you turn left onto the Quarry Trail you will come to a fork in about 150 yards. Take a left and head downhill. After about a third of a mile, the fairly rocky and eroded trail levels out into a smooth dirt trail, and half a mile from the fork the two trails meet up again just past where a short spur trail leads down to the water for a view of the Maumelle River. Shortly after reaching this point, the trail heads uphill and becomes fairly steep.

On your way up the hillside, look for an old car along the trail. After about a quarter mile of uphill you will reach an old road. The Quarry Trail follows the road to the left. If you follow the road to the right instead, you will pass a small quarry on the left and eventually exit the park on Norwood Road.

From the intersection with the old dirt road, the Quarry Trail continues for a few hundred yards to an open area with views of Pinnacle Mountain, an old quarry, the Arkansas River, the Maumelle River, and Lake Maumelle. When you are finished exploring the area, head back the way you came. At the bottom of the hill turn left to take the other fork of the trail back. Shortly after crossing three bridges, you will meet up with the other fork of the trail. Head out the way you came in.

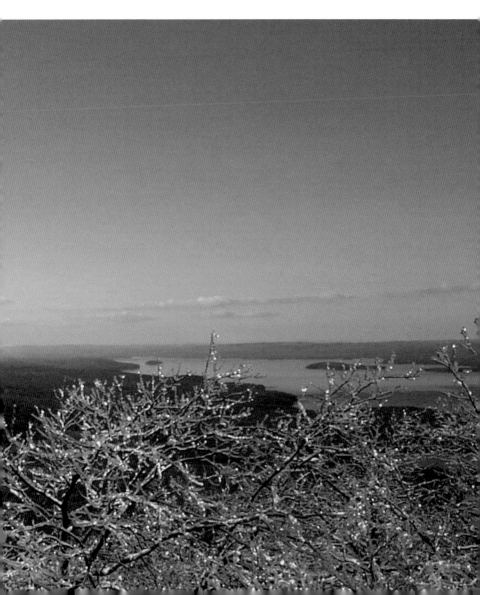

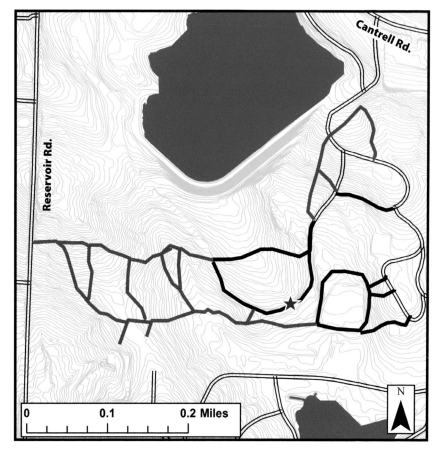

Start/End: 34°46'18.90"N 92°22'10.55"W – Parking Lot west of Baseball Field

Length: 0.75 miles – Loop   **Scenery:** ★★★

Difficulty: Moderate – steep and rocky in places

Reservoir Park is located east of Reservoir Rd. and south of Cantrell Rd. The most attractive part of the park, a large lake that stores drinking water for the city of Little Rock, is currently off-limits and surrounded by barbed wire, however, the park is still home to over a mile of trail, a baseball field, picnic tables, and a basketball court. The best place to catch a glimpse of the lake is from the road on your way in or from the powerline right-of-way along its eastern edge.

The trail starts south of the parking area, near the southwestern corner of the baseball field. From here, the rocky, pine needle covered trail heads west into the woods. The well-worn trail forms a short loop with a network of more primitive trails inside and spurs to nearby homes and roads on the outside.

Since the trail is so short, I encourage you to explore the entire area, but if you stay on the main trail, about a half mile from the baseball field, a spur heads off to the left to Reservoir Rd. where the trail meets a fence that surrounds the lake. Turn right to continue around the loop and stay left at the next several forks to stay on the main trail. After about 350 yards you will reach an old asphalt road. At this point you can take a right and head back to the parking area or take a left to see the lake and explore some of the other trails shown on the map.

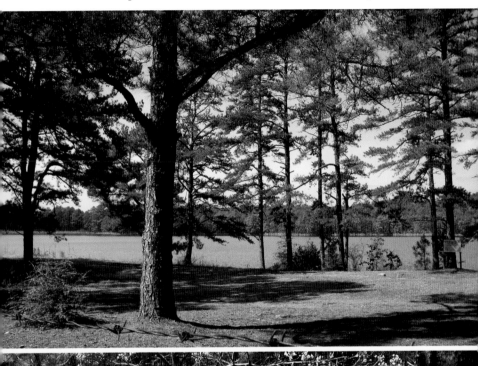

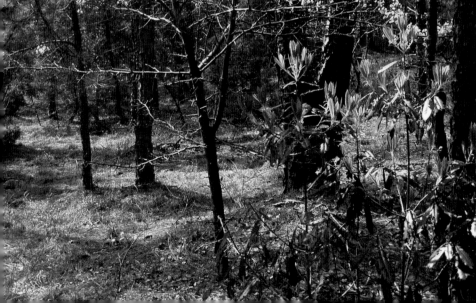

River Mountain Park

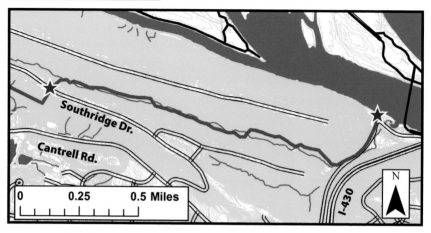

Start: 34°48'1.32"N 92°24'34.76"W - Off Southridge Dr.

End: 34°47'46.20"N 92°23'14.95"W - Off River Mountain Rd.

Length: 1.4 miles – one-way   **Scenery:** ★★★★⚹

Difficulty: Moderate – steep and rocky in places

A very scenic and moderately difficult trail winds its way up the valley, crossing an amazingly beautiful creek many times. There are many interesting features of this creek and perhaps the most unique and stunning is where it flows in a perfectly straight line for hundreds of feet bounded on one bank by a high sheer rock wall.

You can park either along the River Mountain Road in a gravel pull-off area or farther away at the parking lot on the Arkansas River where people put in boats or hit the River Trail. The trail is harder to find from this entrance but starts with the uphill, leaving you with the option to turn around an head downhill whenever you get tired. The trail is easier to find at its upstream entrance where a powerline crosses Southridge in the Walton Heights neighborhood. Park at the crossing and head north along the power line right-of-way. The trail is well-marked with orange diamond blazes (and the old white rectangular ones too). The trail heads down through a beautiful valley paralleling a small stream. The spring is a great time to hike this trail, since it is home to numerous dogwoods. The rocky valley slopes are covered in pines, hickories, oaks, and ironwood trees among others. If you explore off trail, higher up on the slopes you can find some Blackjack oaks as well. As you descend, ferns, mayapples, red maples, and dogwoods become more common. The trail crosses the creek in numerous places and can be fairly difficult at times. As you near River Mountain Road (at about the 1.2 mile mark), the trail curves to the left and heads out to the road.

A short walk down River Mountain Road takes you to the River Trail (pg. 100) near the bridge to Two Rivers Park(pg. 122).

From the pullout on Southridge, heading across the street to the south and following the powerline takes you to Conner Park (pg. 52) and provides nices views of West Little Rock and Chenal Mountain.

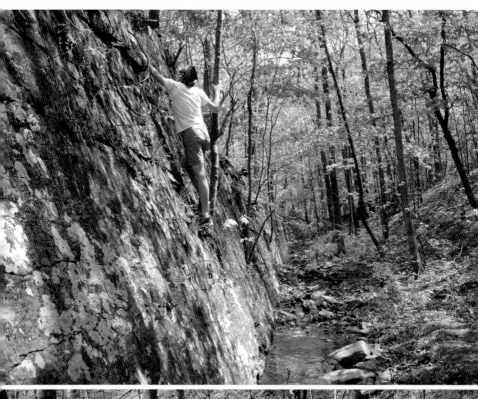

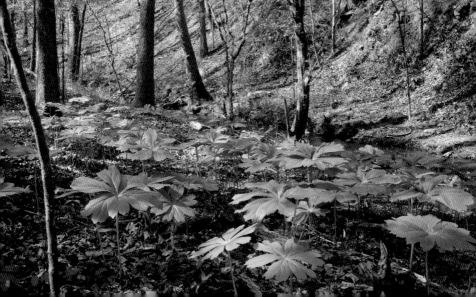

River Trail

The River Trail is a paved bike/pedestrian trail that runs along both the North Little Rock and Little Rock sides of the Arkansas River. Parking for the trail can be found at numerous locations along the trail including:

1. Under I-430 on River Mountain Rd.

2. Cooks Landing in North Little Rock

3. Burns Park in North Little Rock

4. Murray Park on Rebsamen Rd.

5. Rebsamen Park on Rebsamen Rd.

6. At the Big Dam Bridge on Rebsamen Rd.

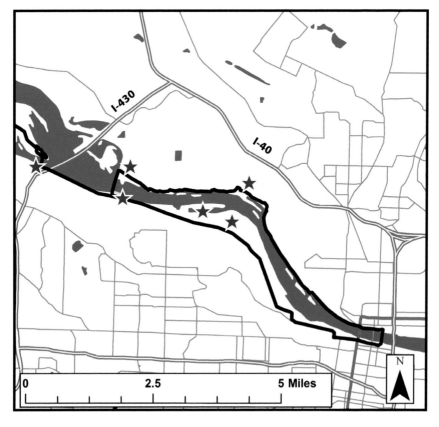

The following pages contain descriptions of the different sections of the trail and then details on traveling the main loop.

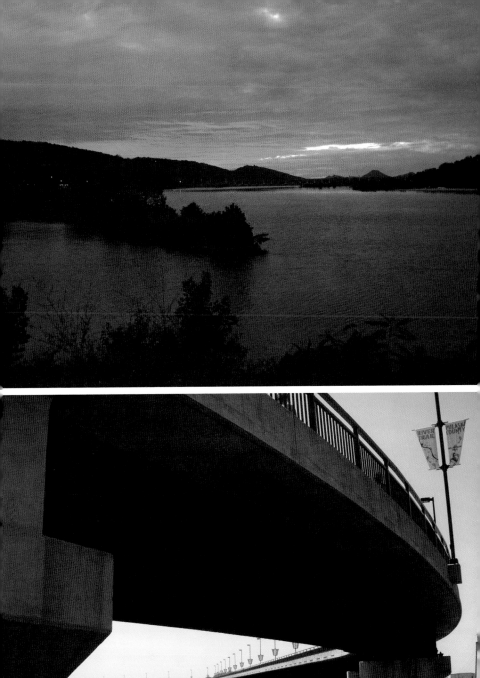

River Trail West

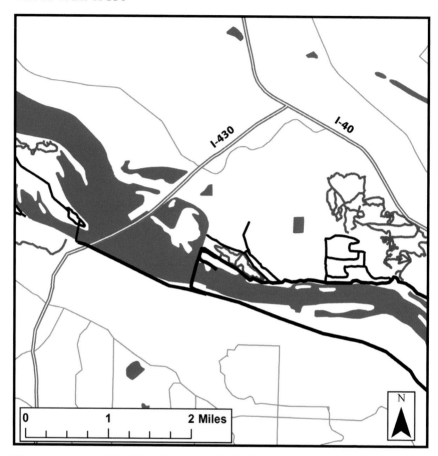

The western end of the River Trail is probably the most scenic and most popular section of the trail. There are multiple spurs off of the main trail in this area. One goes to Two Rivers Park (pg. 122), another up through River Mountain Park (pg. 98), others to Northshore Dr, and another, the Pfieffer Loop, is a dirt trail through the woods for horses, bikers, and hikers. The area around the dam and the Big Dam Bridge is also home to several popular fishing spots.

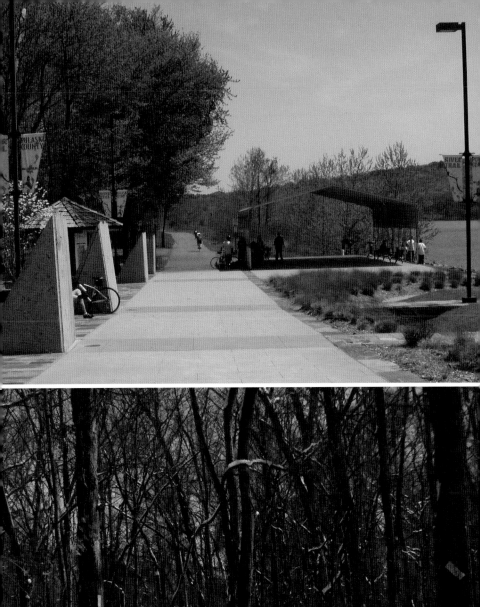
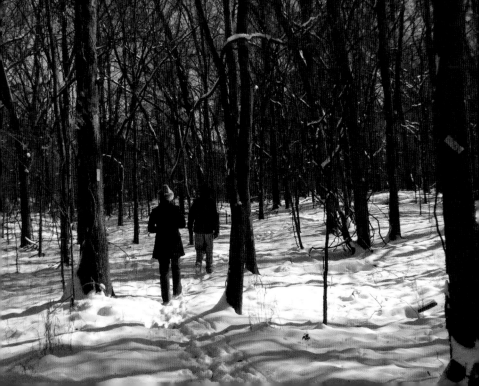

River Trail Central

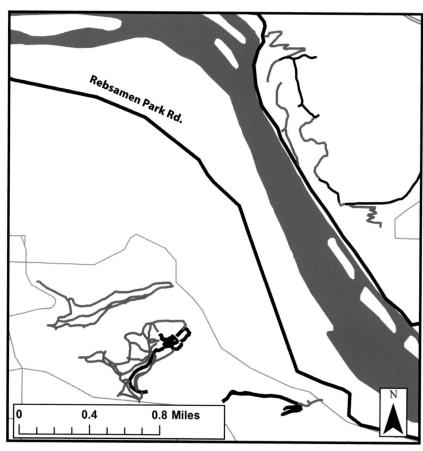

On the North Little Rock side, the trail runs along the river and is quite scenic. It passes by and connects to the Emerald Park trails (pg. 56). On the Little Rock side, much of the trail is just a bike lane on roads with no view of the river. The River Trail passes near Knoop Park (pg. 62) and Allsopp Park (pg. 15).

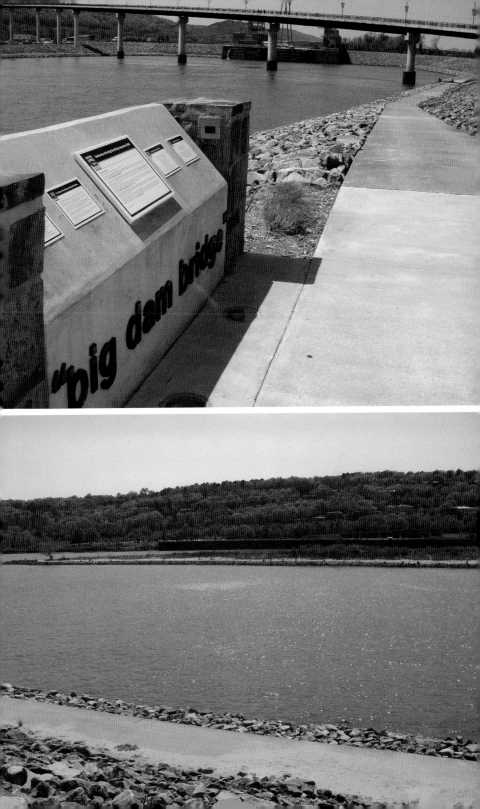

River Trail East

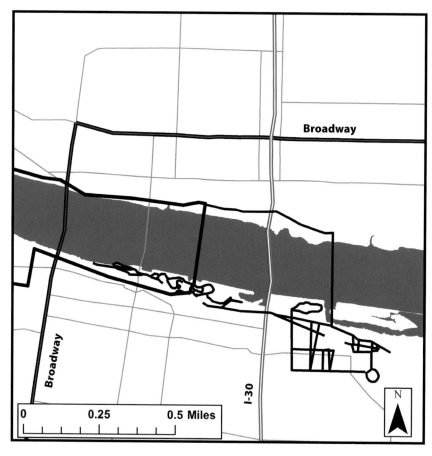

This section of trail connects the downtowns of North Little Rock and Little Rock. There are multiple options for crossing the river here. The Little Rock portion of the trail in this area is the main weak point of the entire River Trail. The trail is virtually non-existent east of Riverdale and through most of downtown as bikers are forced to share the road with cars as they wind their way through a maze of roads with little scenic value. There are several reasons the trail doesn't just continue along the river in this section, but they all boil down to money.

If you have extra time, check out the trails near the Medical Mile, Clinton Library, and Heifer International. They look like children's scribbles on the map above, but are quite scenic in person.

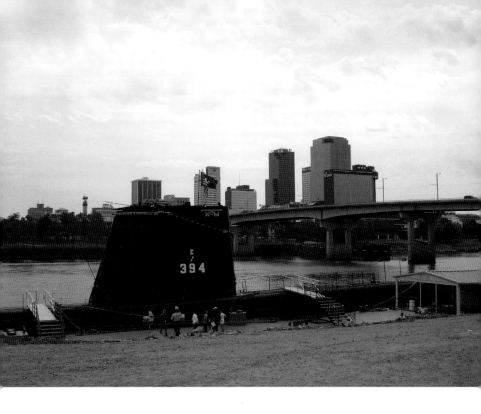

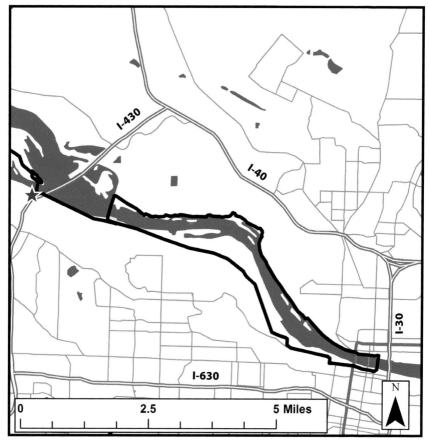

Start/End: 34°47'43.61"N 92°22'38.45"W

Length: 16.25 miles – Loop   **Scenery:** ★★★★✦

Difficulty: Easy – paved and flat

To reach the parking lot at River Mountain Road, take Cantrell west, and turn right on River Mountain Road at its intersection with Cantrell and Old Rodney Parham Road. Follow the road for about a mile and a half under I- 430 to where it dead ends at the River Trail. Take the trail east for about a mile and then get on the recently completed Big Dam Bridge. Getting to the top of the bridge is probably the hardest part of this trail. Once you get to the top it is mostly flat and downhill from here. Take a break on the bridge and look west to see Two Rivers Park, the Little Maumelle, and Pinnacle Mountain. Sunsets from the bridge can be quite amazing. To the east you can see Rebsamen Park, Burns Park, and the cliffs of Emerald Park. When you come down on the North Little Rock side of the bridge you enter the most scenic section of the trail. The next 4 miles takes you through wooded areas, across Burns Park(pg. 44), and into Emerald Park (pg. 56). There are lots of side trails in Emerald Park that take you to the foot of the beautiful cliffs or even up to the top if you've got energy to spare. The views of downtown Little Rock from the top of Emerald Park are quite impressive.

From here the trail heads into downtown North Little Rock and through their riverfront park. Bicyclists and pedestrians can cross into Little Rock on the Junction Bridge or Rock Island Bridge at the Clinton Library. You can also cross on the Main St. Bridge if you don't mind sharing with cars.

Once in Little Rock, the trail follows city roads for quite a while. If you have extra time and energy, take a detour and checkout the Farmer's Market, the Medical Mile, the new Arkansas Game and Fish Center, Bill Clark Presidential Park Wetland Boardwalk, and Clinton Library.

The trail heads west along the river by a great playground and behind the Statehouse Convention Center before essentially ending at Arch St.

From here the trail currently follows Arch St. to Markham, then takes a right on Cross St. followed by a left onto North St.. The trail runs along Cantrell and then Riverfront Dr., before becoming a real bike/pedestrian trail once again at the intersection of Rebsamen Rd. and Riverfront Dr. This section of the trail should change soon, so be sure to follow signs.

On your right you'll see Rebsamen Golf Course and then Murray Park before reaching the Big Dam Bridge once again and continuing on to the parking lot.

For much of the stretch bordering Murray Park, there is a parrallel trail on the other side of the road that is more shaded, but often less well maintained. This alternate trail winds its way through an often swampy bottomland area with cypress, river birch, sycamore and other trees. This trail is recommended for those on foot looking for less traffic and a bit more nature than the wide, busy, grass-lined main attraction.

More information can be found at http://www.rivertrail.org

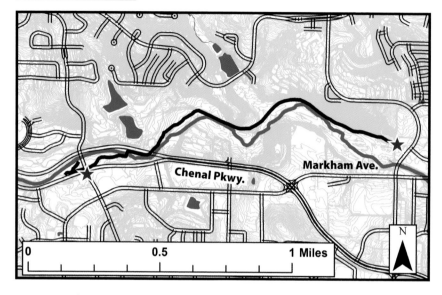

Start: 34°45'16.52"N 92°25'38.90"W

End: 34°45'19.50"N 92°24'25.19"W

Length: 1.4 miles – One-way   **Scenery:** ★★★↲

Difficulty: Easy – paved and flat

Though there are many sections of trail along Rock Creek, that will hopefully one day all be connected, the section I'm calling "Rock Creek Trail" refers solely to the trail in West Little Rock that runs between Loyola Dr. and Bowman Rd. For information on other sections of the trail along Rock Creek go to the Boyle Park trails section of this book (pg. 28).

This trail begins at the southern intersection of Loyola Dr. and Chenal Pkwy. You can park at the gas station or along the shoulder on Chenal if you are brave! The other entrance is located behind the shopping center at Bowman and Markham Place Dr. which has plenty of parking.

Starting from Loyola, the trail heads into the woods and parallels Rock Creek. Much of this section of the creek has been heavily "maintained" and isn't too scenic. However, once you pass under Chenal Parkway you will enter a more natural section of the trail where things have been less disturbed. There are several great views of the creek along this part of the trail and be on the lookout for beautiful tupelo stands.

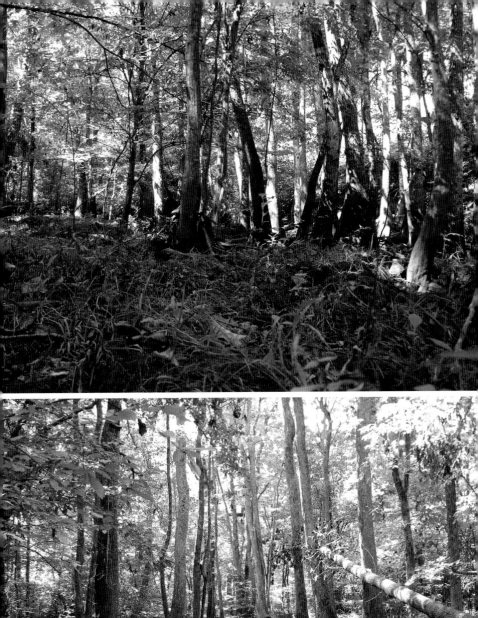
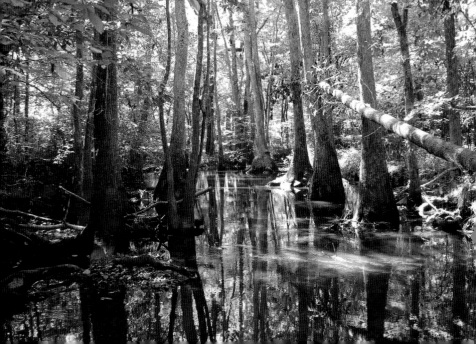

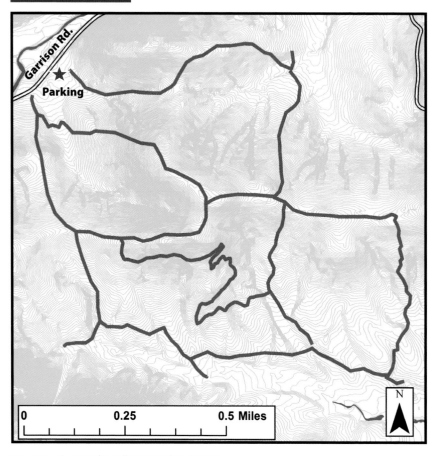

Start/End: 34°49'2.19"N 92°33'51.95"W

Length: 3.0 miles – Loop   **Scenery:** ★★★★

Difficulty: Hard – Trails are steep, rocky, and eroded in many places

Section 13 is a large city park that covers roughly 600 acres (hence the name) off of Garrison Rd. west of Ferndale. This fairly young park is not yet developed, and most of the trails here are just preexisting dirt roads that have not been maintained and are in pretty bad shape. Numerous small streams cross and often run in these roads. Thanks in part to the presence of clay, the trails stay wet for a while after a rain so bring appropriate footwear.

If you want to attempt to get lost in a city park, despite having a book with a map in it, try following the small trail in the center of the park with the switchbacks. If you lose the trail, just head in one direction until you reach one of the larger trails that surround this one.

To hike the outer loop, begin at the trailhead near the entrance to the parking lot off of Garrison (there are two other unmarked trailheads at the northeast and southeast corners of the big field). From here the trail heads south up an incline into the woods. After about 350 yards you will pass a rustic picnic area off to the right. Keep heading uphill and soon you will come to a small opening and a fork in the trail. Turn right to stay on the outer loop.

The trail heads downhill for about 350 yards before leveling out at another fork. Take left to stay on the outer loop. After a quarter-mile, you will see a less-worn trail split off to the right. A short detour here will take you to a small scenic creek. The main trail is level and continues for another 500 or so yards in an area surrounded by dense pine before reaching a nice opening and another fork.

Stay right to continue on the outer loop. From here the trail heads gradually downhill for about 350 yards before coming to another fork at the southeast corner of the park. Take a left and head uphill to stay on the outer loop. Here the forest quickly transitions from dense pine to a mixture of mostly young hardwoods with some pine. Over the next half mile the trail gains 130 feet in elevation before reaching a ridge and yet another fork. Take a left to stay on the outer loop.

Follow the trail (which is in relatively good shape here) west along the ridge for about 500 yards. At the next two forks stay/turn right. From here the trail heads north and downhill for about 500 yards. Stay left at the fork and follow the trail uphill for a quarter-mile. From where the trail levels out, it is just 0.4 mi. down the rocky, eroded trail to the large field and back to the parking lot.

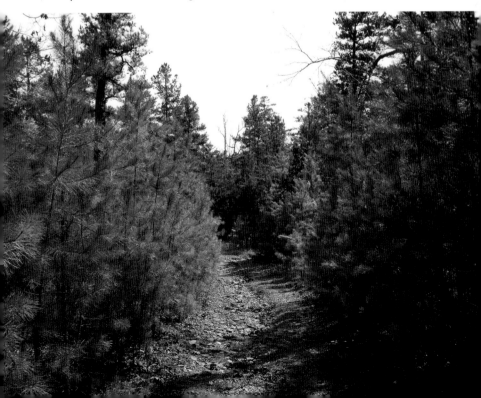

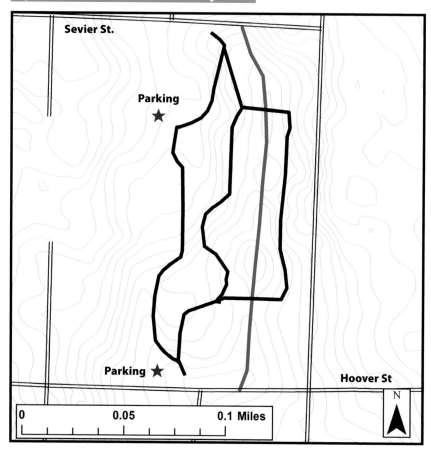

Start: 34°33'39.58"N 92°34'34.71"W

Length: 0.4 miles – Outer Loop   **Scenery:** ★★★

Difficulty: Easy – Padded concrete and fairly flat

Located in Benton, near the intersection of Border St. and Hoover St., the Nelson Rainey trail in Tyndall Park forms a double-loop. This seven foot-wide padded concrete trail meanders through a well-manicured area featuring an amphitheater, creek, and playground. There are a handful of larger oaks and pines along the trail, and a few more young cypress, willow oaks, magnolias, and maples. Parking is located along Hoover St. and Sevier St.

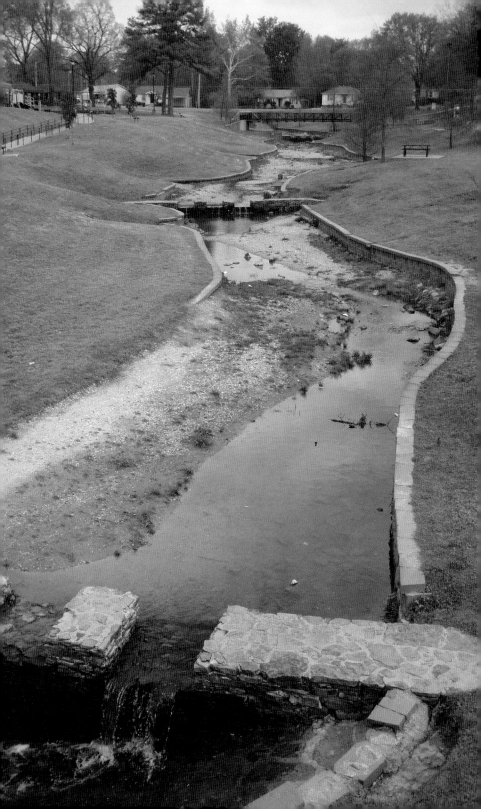

Toltec Mounds State Park

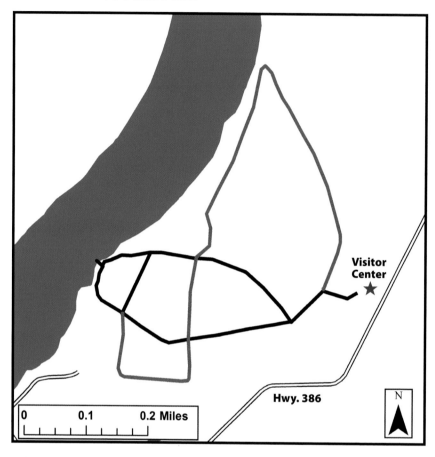

Toltec Mounds State Park is located on Hwy. 386, just off Hwy. 165, between Scott and Keo, southeast of Little Rock. The park gets its name from the large mounds on the site built by the Plum Bayou Culture more than a thousand years ago. The visitor center, where you pay admission, has a small informative museum and restrooms. Be sure to pick up some trail guides before starting your walk.

Two trails, both flat, one paved and the other grass/dirt, loop through the property and take visitors past several large mounds and out to a scenic boardwalk along an oxbow. While the archaeologically significant mounds may be the highlight for many adults, the turtle/fish food dispenser on the boardwalk is usually a big hit with kids.

The park is not open on Mondays. Hours and other information can be found at: http://www.arkansasstateparks.com/toltecmounds/

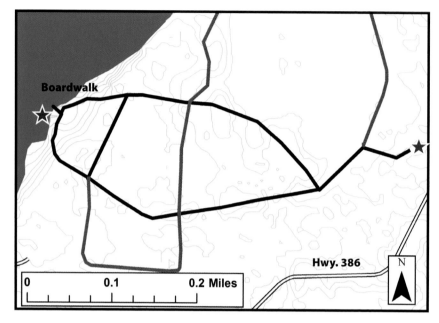

Start: 34°38'44.85"N 92° 3'37.61"W

Length: 1.0 miles – Loop   **Scenery:** ★★★★

Difficulty: Easy – paved and flat

This one mile paved trail begins behind the visitor center. After roughly 200 feet, follow the paved trail as it veers left. In another hundred yards, the trail forks. Both end up at the same place, but stay left to follow the trail marker order and this description.

In 350 yards you will cross the unpaved Plum Bayou trail, and come to Mound C, a short mound with a rounded top, that served as a burial mound. Over the next 175 yards you will approach the two main highlights of the trail, a 50 foot mound and the scenic boardwalk behind it along the cypress-lined oxbow. The boardwalk is partially shaded by ash, sugarberry, maple, elm, persimmon, and cypress trees, making this a good place to take a break in the summer. A turtle/fish food dispenser will happily accept your quarters and give you some pellets to throw to the waiting fish and turtles below. It is not uncommon for over a dozen red eared sliders to congregate under the pier.

When you are finished feeding turtles and looking for snakes hiding amongst the cypress knees, continue around the boardwalk for about 175 yards to Mound B, the second tallest mound in the park. From there it is a short 500 yards back to the visitor center along the paved trail. If you aren't quite ready to leave, or would like to see more of the site, take a left or right onto the unpaved Plum Bayou Trail (pg. 120).

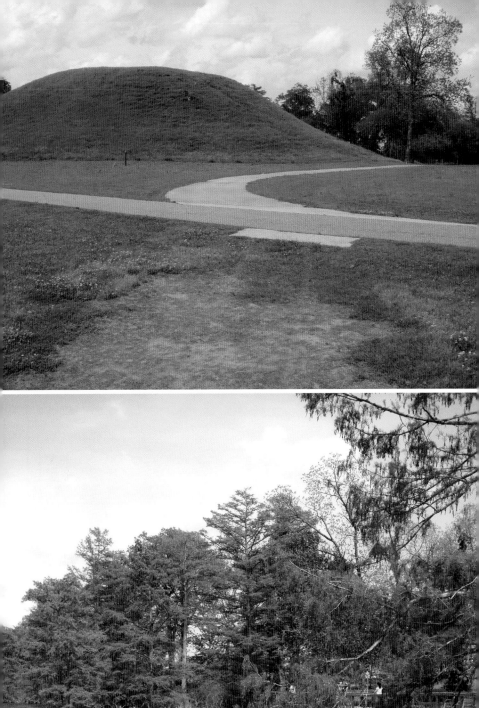

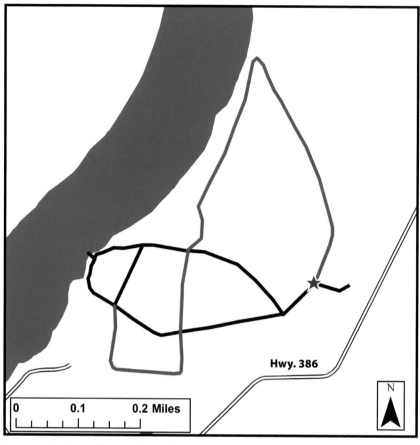

Start: 34°38'44.85"N 92° 3'37.61"W

Length: 1.6 miles – Double-loop   **Scenery:** ★★★★

Difficulty: Easy – dirt/grass and flat

This mile and a half trail begins behind the visitor center where it splits from the paved trail and heads north through the area where the old embankment wall and ditch used to be. As it nears Mound Lake, the trail makes a sharp left and passes by the site of more destroyed earthworks. About 1200 yards from the visitor center, the trail passes Mound B and crosses the Knapp Trail twice before passing under some shady cottonwoods. A remaining section of the embankment wall is just off to the south from here. After looking around and enjoying the shade, follow the trail to where it intersects the paved Knapp Trail. From here it is about a half mile back to the Visitor Center or slightly longer if you go via the boardwalk off to the left.

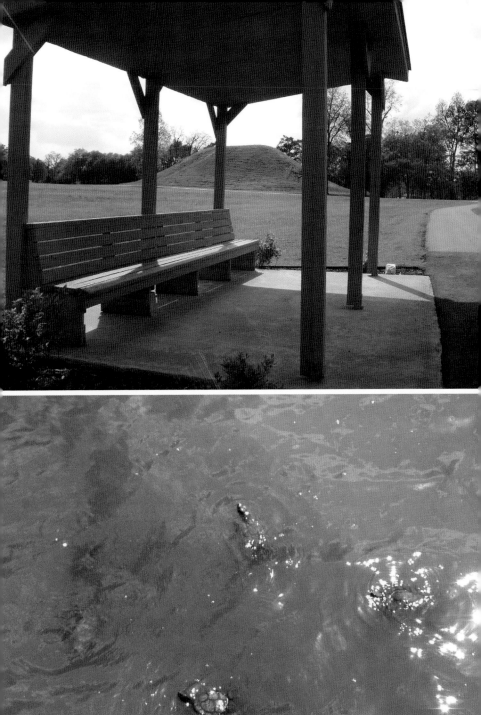

Two Rivers Park

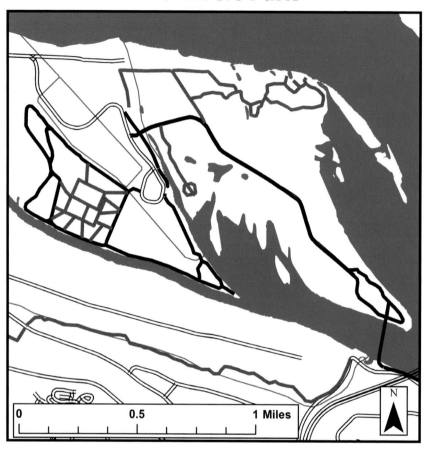

Two Rivers Park in West Little Rock, is one of the city's newer parks. With miles of paved, gravel, and grassy trails as well as a canoe launch providing easy access to the Little Maumelle and Arkansas Rivers, Two Rivers Park has something for everyone from toddlers tricycling on one of the flat paved trails to kayakers looking for a long all day paddle to Pinnacle Mountain and back. The loop out to the eastern end of the park and the two unpaved trails connected to it are somewhat shaded and surrounded by dense vegetation ranging from scrubby forest to swamp to open grassland. The trails in the western part of the park are much more open as they wind through the Garden of Trees and along the Little Maumelle River (pg. 136).

The equestrian trail is grassy and shouldn't be attempted on foot during tick season unless you want to test your tick counting abilities.

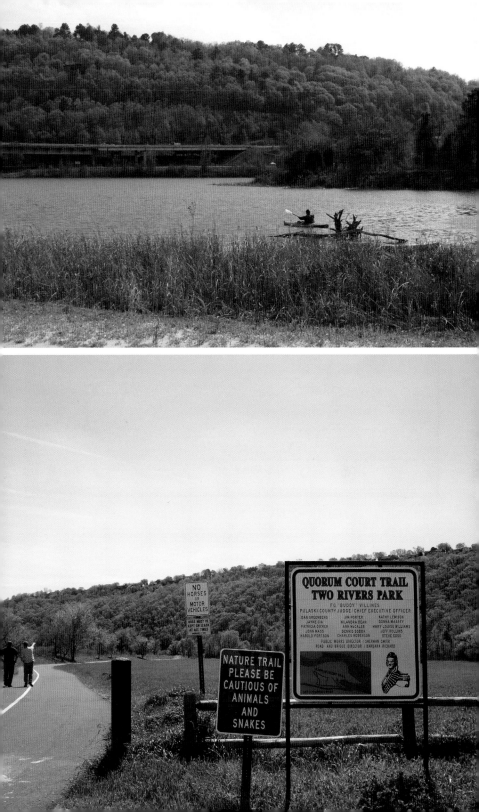

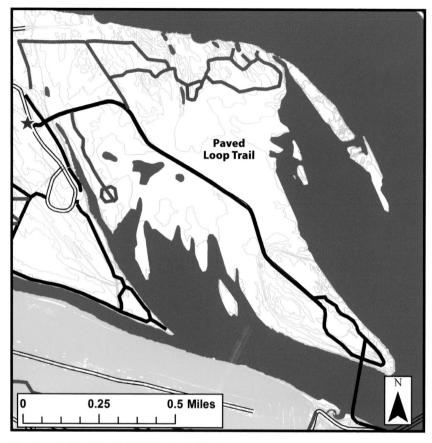

Start/End: 34°48'41.44"N 92°24'6.31"W

Length: 3.0 miles – Loop   **Scenery:** ★★★★

Difficulty: Easy – paved and flat

This flat, paved semi-loop trail is great for a short jog or easy bike ride. It offers interesting views of a variety of habitats including swamp, bottomland hardwood forest, grassland, and pine forest. The trail begins across the road from the second parking lot on your right about half a mile into the park. You will briefly pass through a swampy section before the trail opens up into a large grassy area where it is not uncommon to spot large numbers of deer. A short grassy side trail leads off to your right.

As you continue down the paved trail, you will encounter more wetland areas with lots of horsetail growing along the trail. After about a mile the trail splits to form a short loop. To the left you will enter a dense pine stand. To the right there is an open grassy area.

At the far end of the trail treat yourself to some great views of the Arkansas River and the I-430 bridge. There are picnic tables for anyone who feels like carrying supplies this far.

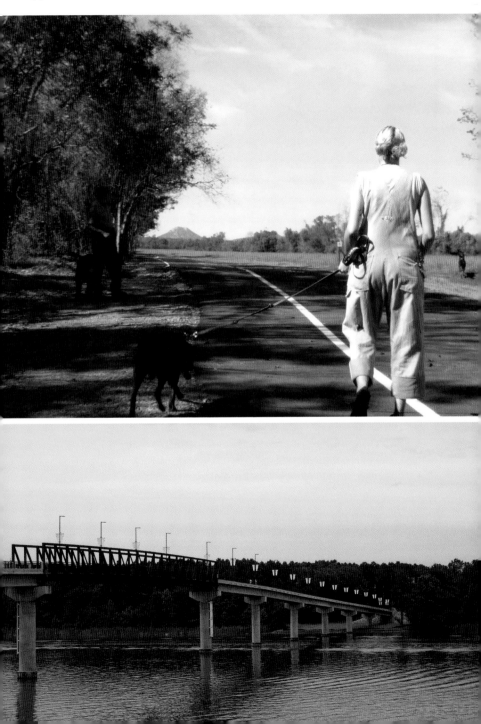

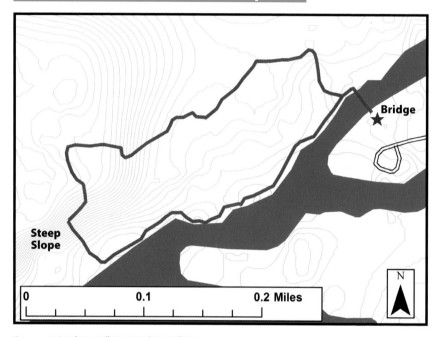

Start: 34°26'54.60"N 92° 6'58.05"W

Length: 0.75 miles – Loop   **Scenery:** ★★★✦

Difficulty: Moderate – steep in places

Tar Camp Park is located on River Rd. roughly five miles east of Redfield. The park has dozens of campsites and picnic tables along the Arkansas River in addition to a playground, boat launch, and the White Bluff Nature Trail.

The trail is in the western part of the park near several popular fishing spots along a backwater of the Arkansas River. Park near the big red bridge. Once you cross the bridge, turn left and you'll find a map of the trail.

Just past the map, the trail forks. To the left it is a flat, thin, dirt path along the water. Take the trail to the right, which heads into the woods. The path here is well-worn. As you head gradually uphill, large oaks tower over smaller dogwoods. The ground is home to mayapples and muscadine vines. The trail follows the bluff line for awhile and then abruptly drops down the side of the bluff. The map shows steps at this point, but at the time this was written, there appeared to have been a landslide (or at least no steps and a pile of wood at the bottom of the bluff). At this point you can turn back and return the way you came, or make your way down the steep slope.

At the base of the bluff, follow the trail for 200 feet to the backwater of the Arkansas River and turn left. Sycamore, sweetgum, sugarberry, box elders, and large cottonwoods dominate this section of the trail, which is unmarked, overgrown in places, and less well-worn. At a few spots along the way, you can spot the smokestack of the White Bluff coal power plant just two miles to the southwest. From here, it is a short, flat walk along the shore back to the bridge and parking area.

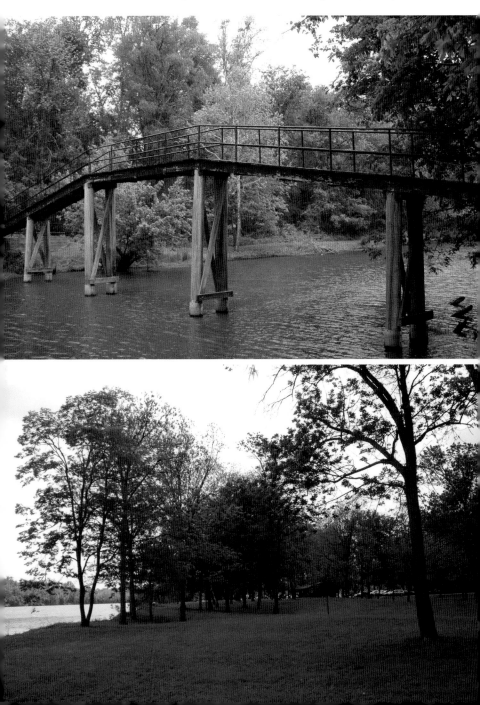

Water Trails

In addition to having a wide selection of trails for hiking, biking, and horseback riding, Central Arkansas is also home to several great water trails. With the Arkansas River in the center, the Saline, Maumelle, and Little Maumelle to the west, Cadron to the north, and Fourche Creek in the Little Rock area, residents are never far from a great place to paddle.

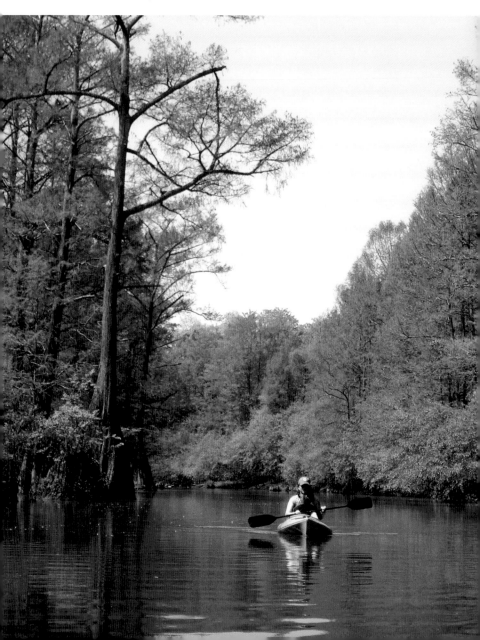

Fourche Creek

Fourche Creek is the probably the least floated of the options mentioned above, though it is perhaps the most conveniently located for people living in Little Rock. It flows past numerous public parks including: Otter Creek Park, Hindman Park, Benny Craig, Fourche Bottoms, Interstate Park, the Audubon Nature Center, and Remmel Park. There are developed launches at Hindman Park, Benny Craig Park, Interstate Park and Remmel Park.

Though it is relatively short, Fourche Creek flows through three of Arkansas' six major ecoregions. Over a day-long float the scenery changes from a gravel-bottom stream lined with river birch, box elder, and sycamore to a highly sinuous silt-bottomed creek lined with large cypress and silver maples.

This unique creek gives paddlers a taste of scenic wilderness while providing frequent reminders that you are actually in the state's most populous city.

Much more information on the creek can be found at:
http://www.fourchecreek.org

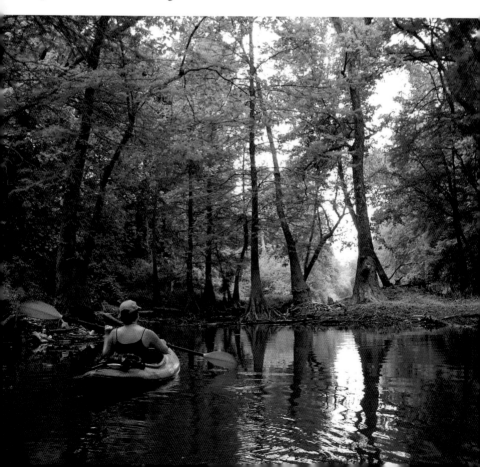

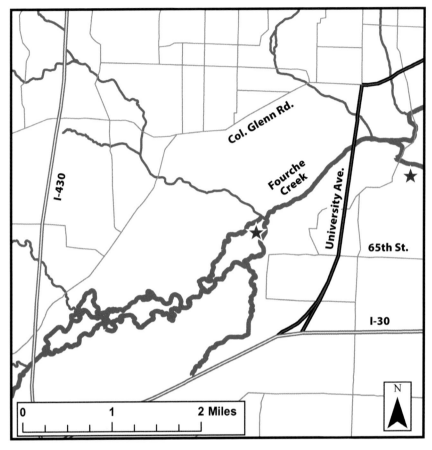

Start: 34°41'46.38"N 92°21'39.23"W (Hindman Park)

Finish: 34°42'10.09"N 92°19'36.60"W (Benny Craig Park)

Length: 2.4 mi. - One way   **Scenery:** ★★★↙

Difficulty: Moderate – depending on flow you might have to portage frequently

Though this section is labeled as starting at I-430, this description begins with putting in at Hindman Park. Launching near I-430 either at the Highway Department or across the creek at the nursery can be tricky, but is definitely worth it. That section of the creek is quite scenic and completely devoid of other people. Of note for plant people, the banks of Fourche Creek in this area are home to the very rare Arkansas Meadow-rue.

A much easier place to put-in in this section is Hindman Park, located at the west end of 65th St. If you want to float upstream on Fourche it is best to park on the gravel shoulder near the southern entrance to the park and put-in near the rock vane that has been constructed in the creek. If you are looking to float down to Benny Craig, you might want to put in a little further downstream at the bridge.

From the bridge paddle downstream past the north end of the golf course. Spotted gar and green herons are pretty common in this area. After about a quarter mile, the creek leaves the power line right of way and enters a forested stretch. There is often a several foot high beaver dam around this point that can be ramped over, or for the less adventurous, portaged around. The creek is fairly straight and scenic for the next three quarters of a mile. Look for some large cypress with dozens of knees! Of possible side interest to geology buffs, one of the easternmost outcroppings of novaculite (found in the Ouachita Mountains) can be found along the steep hillside to your right.

At the one mile mark, the creek enters an unsightly stretch where it has been channelized and dredged for flood control and to protect University Ave. When passing under the bridge, be on the lookout for swallows, which can put on quite a show for intruders at certain times of the year. After about half a mile, Rock Creek, the largest tributary of Fourche, pours into the creek on the left. The creek then heads into the woods again. After ~0.1 miles, Fourche Creek forks. Take the channel to the right, which is usually the only branch with much water in it. Be sure you take the correct route since these forks of the creek don't come back together for over 6 miles!

As the creek gradually turns to the right, you might see a man-made pond just over the bank to your right. The creek connects to this pond, but I don't recommend making a side trip into it. Just past the 2-mile mark, you pass under Mabelvale Pike. Just past the bridge you may have to portage around a yellow trash boom. From here, the canoe launch at Benny Craig park is a short straight half mile trip with BFI landfill on your left and the launch coming up on your right. If you pass under a railroad bridge you've gone about a quarter-mile too far! Benny Craig Park is located near the intersection of Gum Springs Rd. and Rosemoor Dr.

Middle Section: Benny Craig Park - Interstate Park

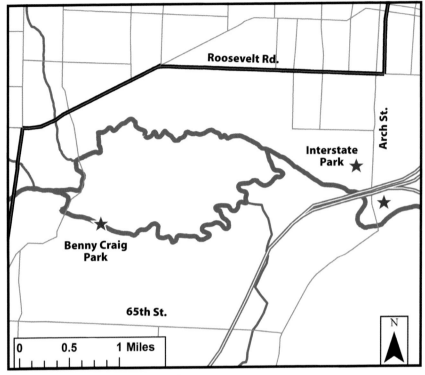

Start: 34°42'10.09"N 92°19'36.60"W

Finish: 34°42'29.05"N 92°17'6.36"W

Length: 4.4 mi. - One way   **Scenery:** ★★★★✦

Difficulty: Moderate – depending on flow you might have to portage frequently

Easily the most frequently floated section of Fourche Creek, the middle section is where great scenery and ideal water depth overlap. Official concrete put-ins can be found at Benny Craig Park and Interstate Park. Unlike many popular floating destinations around the state, the mile and a half stretch of Fourche Creek upstream of Interstate Park is floatable year-round with no scraping or portaging. A highly recommended and more detailed map of this section can be found at: http://www.fourchecreek.org/Floating.html.

The launch at Benny Craig Park, located near the intersection of Gum Springs Rd. and Rosemoor Dr., is a very short walk north from the parking lot. Follow the creek to your right to head downstream, where just past the park you will pass under an active railroad bridge. A few minutes later you will reach an elevated gas pipeline that you may have to portage around. After three quarters of a mile, you will come to a sharp bend in the creek with concrete all over the right bank.

During low flow be careful not to scrape your boat on the concrete.

Shortly after you pass the concrete banks, you will come upon an elevated sewer line. Since all the landmarks I've mentioned so far might sound ugly, I feel compelled to mention that this section of the creek is actually quite scenic with cypress, silver maples, and box elder lining the banks. That said, due to the creek's size and sinuosity, unsightly trash tends to pile up in large mats at multiple locations along this stretch of the creek. This is a problem that Audubon Arkansas and the City of Little Rock are working on, but one that will likely take decades to solve.

After a little over 2 miles you will come to the first of three large power line crossings. At the 3 mile mark, the creek begins to widen after you pass by the third large power line crossing. After a couple large bends, the creek becomes wider and fairly straight and deep for the last 1 mile leg to Interstate Park. The one exception involves a difficult to spot sharp left turn you will need to make about a half mile upstream of the takeout at 34°42'39.62"N 92°17'38.34"W. Hopefully this spot will be marked with an "Arkansas Water Trails" sign by the time this book is in print. However, if you happen to find yourself at a dead end, you've passed the turn and need to backtrack about 100 yards and look for your turn. If you hate backtracking you can always just portage 40 to 50 yards to the east and meet back up with the creek.

From here it is a short, easy float to Interstate Park. You'll know you are getting close when you reach the wooden railroad bridge. To give you some idea of how high flood waters can get here, I've seen a large dead tree stuck about 9 feet up on the bridge! About 120 yards past the bridge is the takeout at the southern edge of Interstate Park.

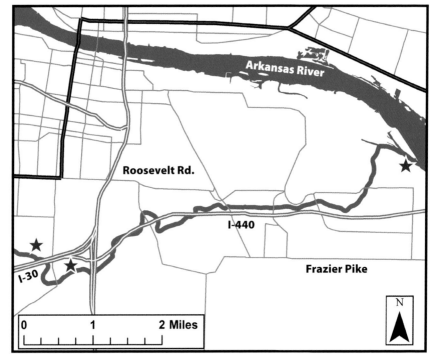

Start: 34°42'29.05"N 92°17'6.36"W

Finish: 34°43'34.72"N 92°11'16.51"W

Length: 7.6 mi. - One way   **Scenery:** ★★★↲

Difficulty: Moderate – depending on flow you might have to portage some.

This float begins at Interstate Park and heads downstream. This is an interesting float but overall, not the most classically scenic. Since much of the route is wide and deep, this section can be much busier than areas upstream. Be ready to share the creek with motorboats and jet skis. Interstate 440 and the airport are never far away, making this the noisiest section of the creek to float.

Immediately after leaving the canoe launch, you will pass under a power line and then under Interstate 30. The next 1200 yards are the most scenic of the float. The creek is narrow and surrounded by cypress. A short distance from the creek explorers can find numerous beaver dams on small side streams and large cypress trees with seven foot knees!

After passing under Arch Street, the creek immediately widens. Although not easily seen from the water, there is an old home foundation on the north side of the creek in this section. About half a mile past the bridge, a small cypress knee lined channel connects the creek to a large pond that is accessible from Arch St. and has a parking area.

Less then 175 yards past the entrance to the borrow pond, the creek passes under Interstate 530. The next half mile is perfectly straight where the railroad cuts off a stretch of the original channel of Fourche Creek forming an oxbow lake that is part of the Audubon Arkansas Nature Center. If you pay close attention, you can find where the oxbow drains under the railroad. A rough portage under the railroad and over a large beaver dam will provide you with a nice side-float on the scenic lake.

Continuing on the main (straightened) channel of the creek you will pass by a large borrow pond to the north and then under I-440 several times over the next three quarters of a mile.

At the 2.7 mile mark, the trail passes under Springer Blvd. and loses most of its natural character for the rest its path to the Arkansas River. Just before you pass under Springer and bid farewell to scenic tree-lined sections of the creek, look for an odd cylindrical brick structure on the north side of the creek. Feel free to e-mail me if you have some good guesses as to what it was used for.

During the first half mile downstream of Springer Blvd. you will pass under multiple highway on-ramps and off-ramps and I-440. The drastically altered channel then widens to about 150 feet. Over the next 3 miles, the creek passes under I-440, a railroad bridge, Airport Road, and Lindsey Road before reaching the boat launch at Remmel Park (34°43'0.69"N 92°12'23.71"W). This makes a good put-in or take out spot as there are no developed launches further downstream. Half a mile downstream of Remmel Park, you will reach the last place where it might be feasible to take-out or put-in, at Fourche Dam Pike. Along this road, near the creek, there is a Civil War plaque, marking the Engagement at Fourche Bayou that occurred on September 10, 1863. It would be great to see a photograph from this battle, since I'm sure the creek must have looked very different from its current widened, mowed, and rip-rapped state.

From Fourche Dam Pike it is just over a mile to the creek's confluence with the Arkansas River.

Little Maumelle

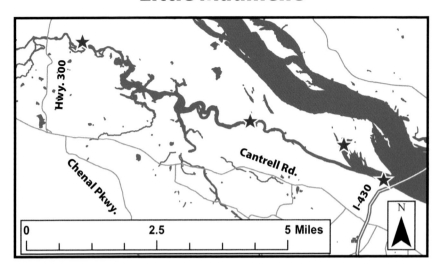

The Little Maumelle is generally regarded as the most scenic float in Little Rock. Over 8 miles of floatable creek offer stunning views of Pinnacle Mountain, dense groves of cypress, cattail stands and the I-430 Bridge. Canoes can be rented at the Pinnacle Mountain Visitor Center.

There are numerous places to put-in along the Little Maumelle including: Pinnacle Mtn. Canoe Launch at east end of parking lot - 34°50'19.08"N 92°29'28.14"W

House on Burnett Road off Pinnacle Valley Road (pay ~$5) 34°48'53.54"N 92°26'26.03"W

Two Rivers Park - 34°48'28.71"N 92°23'55.59"W

Boat Launch/River Trail Access Off River Mountain Rd. - 34°47'55.63"N 92°23'7.06"W

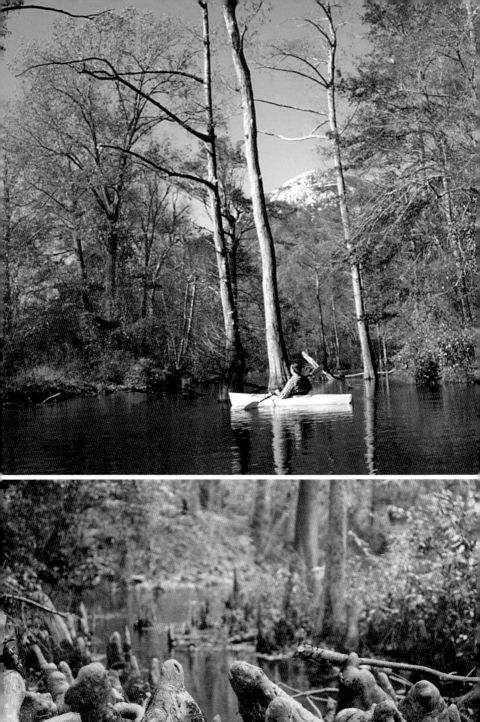
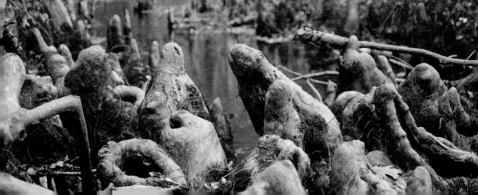

Little Maumelle: Pinnacle Mountain - Two Rivers Park

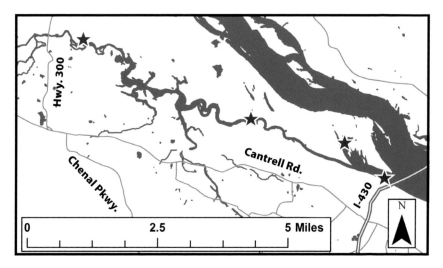

Start: 34°50'19.08"N 92°29'28.14"W

End: 34°48'28.71"N 92°23'55.59"W

Length: 9.0 miles - one-way   **Scenery:** ★★★★★

Starting at the boat launch at the far end of the West Summit parking lot, head downstream (to the left facing the creek). For the first few minutes the creek parallels a branch of the base trail, so wave to any hikers you see. After a quarter mile or so the stream narrows and turns to the left, passing through some cypress knee rapids. If the water is low, you may have to get out and pull you boat through this section. Be sure to keep an eye out for turtles and snakes sunning themselves on trees and logs in the middle of the water. A railroad bridge marks the half-mile point and makes a good turn around point if you are looking for a short float. There isn't usually much of current in the Little Maumelle, so be sure to give yourself plenty of time if you plan to do all nine miles!

Continuing down the trail, you will pass under a high voltage power line. About a mile later, the creek opens up and becomes a bit harder to follow. Several side streams, islands, thick cypress stands and deceiving dead ends make exploring this area a fun but time-consuming task. To stay on track be sure to bring a good map (either in this book, on Google earth, or elsewhere). This trail may now be marked with Arkansas Water Trail blazes, making navigation much easier. One of my favorite parts of the trail is located just past the two mile mark where a dense grove of cypress stands in the channel. Quietly weaving your way through this half-mile section of trail, you can surprise ducks, herons, turtles, snakes, and fishermen in flat-bottom boats. At the 3.5 mile mark, the trail passes under 2 large pipes and then enters three large bends with large islands. Much of the year one side of the islands is impassable due to shallow water and large amounts of vegetation, but those paths less traveled can provide a fun, challenging shortcut under the right conditions. Shortly after you pass under Pinnacle Valley Road, you will see a powerline crossing the creek. At the time this was written, you could pay five dollars to park and put-in or take out at this house located at the end of Burnett Road. Some of the land here has been up for sale, so putting in here may not be an option much longer.

If still open after a recent large flood, another fun place to take-out or at least take a break is the bait shop near Two Rivers Park, located at about the 6 mile mark. Park the kayaks and grab a soda and some snacks from this unique store before embarking on the final leg of the float. For the next 1.5 miles, Two Rivers Park is to your left and a railroad and Walton Heights neighborhood are to your right. When the trail opens up you have the choice of either hanging a sharp left and traveling half a mile to the canoe launch at Two Rivers Park or staying straight, heading towards the I-430 bridge, and taking out at the boat launch located off of River Mountain Road. This parking lot can be used to access the River Trail or River Mountain Trail. The trail is dominated by cypress, but large silver maple, sycamores, river birch, water oaks, and shagbark hickory are also found along the banks. In the spring and summer you will probably see turtles and snakes sunning themselves. Deer occasionally swim across the Little Maumelle. In the summer large blooming lily pads cover huge swathes of the creek

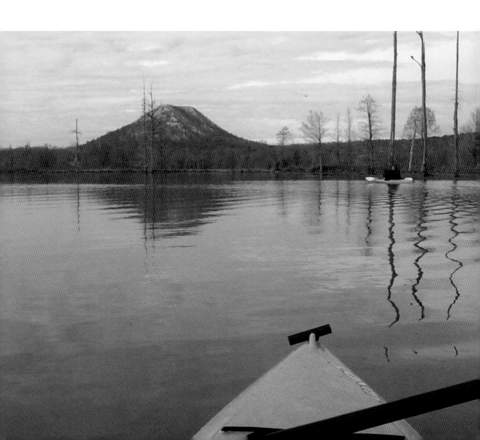

Saline River

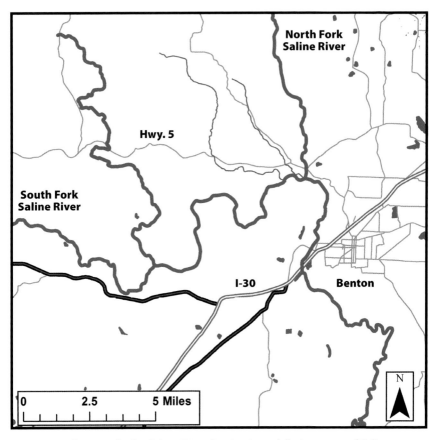

Appropriately enough, the Saline River begins in and drains most of Saline County. From these headwaters, located roughly 25 miles west of Little Rock, the Saline flows over 130 miles south until its confluence with the Ouachita River near the Louisiana border. In Central Arkansas, several branches of the Saline can be accessed for floating and fishing near Benton. The river can be accessed at the following locations:

North Fork Saline River:
Steel Bridge Rd. - 34°39'38.25"N 92°38'7.67"W
Hwy. 5 - 34°36'14.84"N 92°37'4.81"W

Saline River:
Lyle Park - 34°35'13.26"N 92°36'17.33"W
Moore Ford - 34°33'39.30"N 92°41'18.56"W
Peeler Bend - 34°35'6.15"N 92°38'47.59"W
I-30 - 34°33'14.93"N 92°37'17.75"W

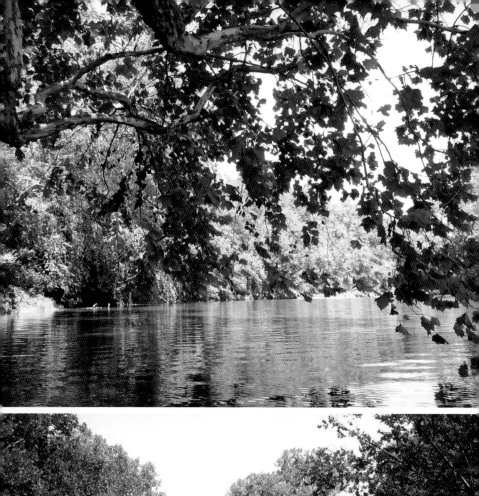
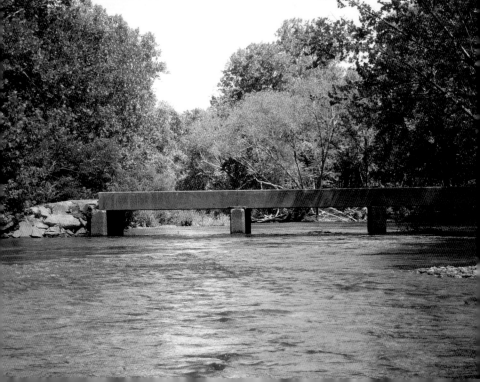

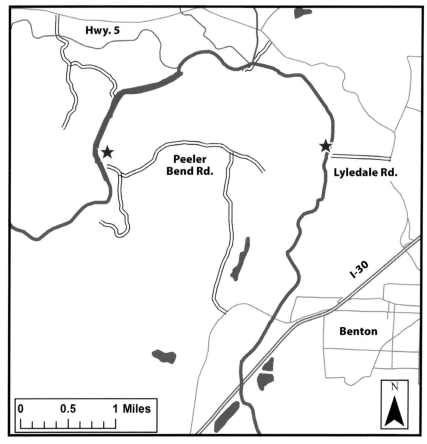

Start: Peeler Bend Rd. - 34°35'6.15"N 92°38'47.59"W

End: Lyle Park - 34°35'13.26"N 92°36'17.33"W

Length: 3.8 miles - one-way   **Scenery:** ★★★★

Difficulty: Easy–short, few tricky parts

The float from Peeler Bend to Lyle Park is a scenic medium to short float. If you are looking for something longer, you can put in further upstream at Moore Ford or take out downstream of Lyle Park at I-30.

Arrange a shuttle with Saline River Canoe or park one car at Lyle Park off Lyledale Rd., and drive the other car back down Hwy. 5 to I-30. Take the highway or frontage road west to the next exit and stay on the frontage road until you reach Hwy. 229. Turn right and in about three quarters of a mile turn right again on Peeler Bend Rd. Follow this road for about 3 miles through a suburban/rural residential area. The road dead-ends at the Peeler Bend boat launch.

The float begins with a paddle through a wide, long mile and a half pool. The river here is lined with leaning sycamore and silver maples, with large hickories and oak in the background. At the end of the pool, a small side stream enters on the left. River birch and bright green watergrass are common on this stretch.

In a half mile willow dominate the banks as the river shrinks even more and speeds up. With the right amount of flow there can be a brief, exciting bit of whitewater here. Another half mile brings you to the confluence with the North Fork.

Important: Just 50 yards downstream of this confluence is a low bridge. If the water is up, this bridge can be dangerous. If this is your first time on the river, it might be a good idea to pull over and study the situation before proceeding.

The river forks a half mile below the bridge, forming a large island. Taking a left, you will pass a large house shortly before the two forks merge. It is another three quarters of a mile down a long pool to the concrete take-out at Lyle Park on the left.

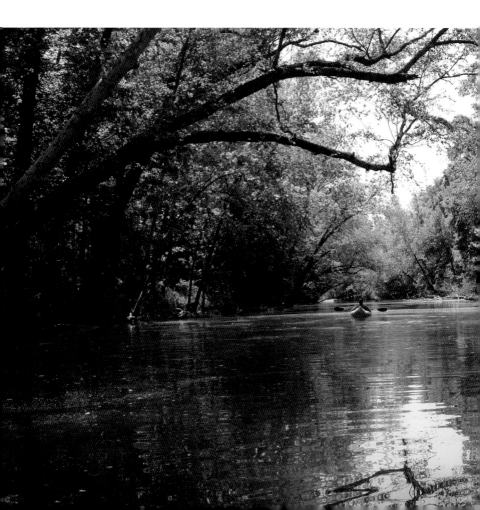

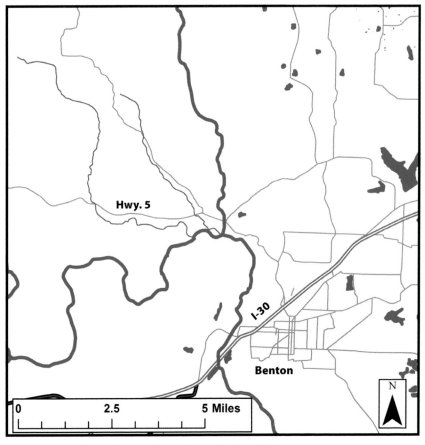

Start: Steel Bridge Rd. - 34°39'38.25"N 92°38'7.67"W

End: Lyle Park - 34°35'13.26"N 92°36'17.33"W

Length: 6.2 miles - one-way   **Scenery:** ★★★★

Difficulty: Easy–short, few tricky parts

The North Fork of the Saline River begins around Paron, AR and merges with the Middle Fork about 20 miles to the southeast. The section described here can be pretty shallow in the summer, so be sure to check the USGS website before starting this one (or just move downstream a little if it looks too low at Steel Bridge Rd.). Ideal gage levels for this stretch are 4-5 feet. The put-in for this float is located 7 miles north of Benton on Steel Bridge Rd., roughly three quarters of a mile west of the intersection with Brazil Rd. and 3 miles west of Congo Ferndale Rd. Park on the gravel along the west side of the bridge and follow the path on the south side of the road down to the water.

From here, the cobble, gravel, and sand-bottomed stream flows south under the shade of leaning sycamore and river birch. Along the way you will also see some silver maple, cypress, and sweet gum along the banks, while tall oaks and hickories can be seen slightly higher up.

After three quarters of a mile, the river begins to curve slightly to the left as it passes a private campsite and, a bit later, a scenic bluff, both on the right side. A pool about 500 yards long begins at the bluff. Hopefully you picked a day when the river has some flow and the wind isn't blowing against you, as this is just one of the first of many long pools on this float.

The next 1.7 miles are fairly scenic, but fallen trees can be a problem. This issue really becomes a problem about a half mile after you pass under the power line. Multiple fallen trees and gravel bars form a tangle that will likely require portaging for some time to come.

Over the next mile, there are long stretches of bedrock where the river is pretty shallow. If you float here with the USGS gauge below 4 feet you may have to walk.

In another 500 yards you will pass under the Hwy. 5 bridge. Just past the bridge is a river access point that is also a popular swimming and fishing spot. If you want to have a shorter float this is a good take-out spot. When water levels are too low to put in upstream, this is a good put-in.

Important: Shortly after the bridge and put-in, the river bends and confluences with the Middle Fork. A bridge with low clearance crosses the river immediately below this point. If the water is high, this bridge is a real hazard. If you haven't floated this section before and the water is moving much at all, you should pull off 400 yards down from the bridge at the bend and visually inspect the bridge before proceeding.

The river forks a half mile below the bridge, forming a large island. If you go left, you will pass a large house on the left shortly before the two forks merge. From here it is three quarters of a mile down a long pool to the concrete take-out which will be on your left.

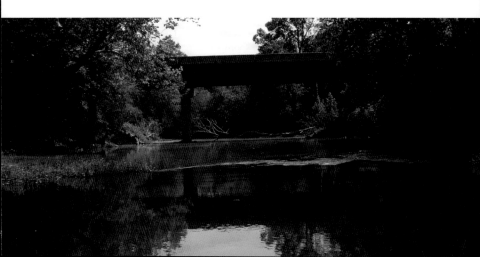

Potential/Upcoming Trails

This section of the book contains information on trails being planned or worked on. If you would like to see more trails built (including the ones on the pages that follow) there are several steps you could take:

1. Work with your neighborhood association to plan, clear, and maintain a trail on public or neighborhood property.

2. Contact your mayor and city board of directors and let them know that you appreciate our parks and trails and would like to see more.

3. Contact the County Judge and let him know you appreciate the county's work on trails and would like to see more built.

4. Contact your state and federal representatives to let them know you support funding for parks and trails projects. There are often projects that have already been approved but the funding has not been appropriated. One example of this is the approved, but so far unfunded, Corps of Engineers project in Fourche Bottoms. If funded completely, this project would include the construction of an access road, boardwalks, and canoe launch in the ~2,000 ac. Fourche Bottoms area in the center of Little Rock.

There is a big push now for improving trail connectivity. Many people want to use trails for more than just recreation and connecting existing trails and trail systems is a great way to provide routes for people to get from home to work or shopping areas without having to drive. The River Trail in Little Rock and North Little Rock is a good example of a trail that is very popular with recreational users and commuters since it connects residential areas to large parks and commercial areas including downtown.

Audubon Nature Center

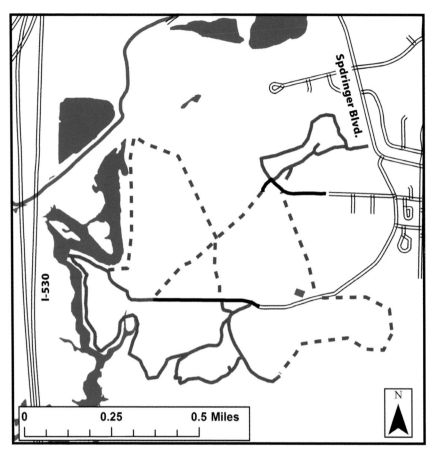

Though two trails at the Nature Center are included in this book, there are many more planned for the park. A trail will eventually run from behind the Nature Center building on Springer Blvd. up the grassy hill and through the woods to connect with the other trails in the park. Other trails there will link to rare nepheline syenite glades that are home to cacti and other unique plants. A canoe launch will be built to improve floating access to the Fourche Creek oxbow lake on the property.

Coleman Creek Greenway Trail

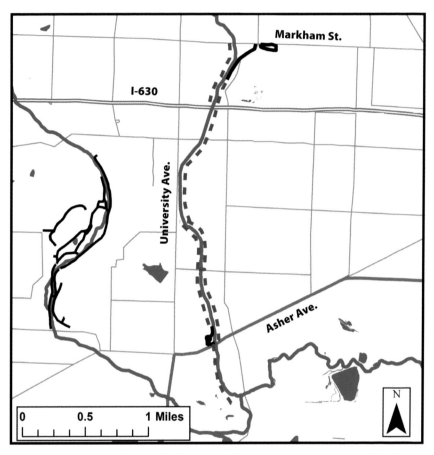

Spanning approximately 3 miles from Markham St. near War Memorial Stadium south to Fourche Creek near Asher Ave. and University Ave., this trail will follow Coleman Creek through War Memorial Park and the UALR Campus. The different sections of this trail are at various levels of the planning and construction process. Some sections in War Memorial Park and at UALR are already in place.

Connecting these two sections initially will likely involve placing bike lanes and larger sidewalks along existing roads, with the hope of placing a dedicated bike/pedestrian trail closer to the creek at a later date.

Fourche Bottoms Trail

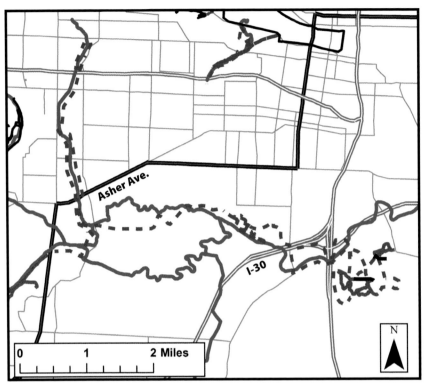

This trail will connect the Coleman Creek Greenway Trail (pg. 148) to the State Fairgrounds, the South End neighborhood, Interstate Park, and the Audubon Nature Center. The planned route runs through one of Little Rock's largest and least developed parks, Fourche Bottoms, which contains two branches of Fourche Creek and several large borrow ponds. The area is home to coyotes, bobcats, beaver, river otters, deer, and many species of waterfowl.

More information on Fourche Bottoms and this trail can be found at:

www.fourchecreek.org

http://www.villagecommonslr.com/

Hindman Future Trails

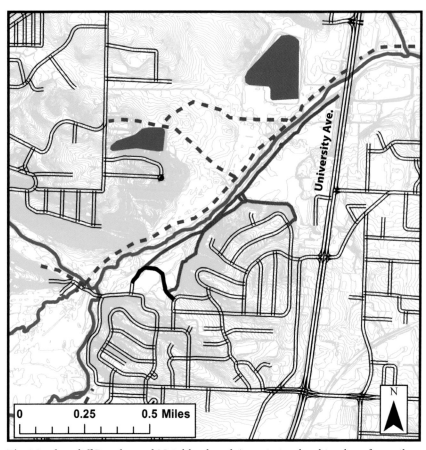

The Meadowcliff Brookwood Neighborhood Association has big plans for trails in Hindman Park. In addition to paving many of the existing unpaved trails, the association plans on connecting these trails to Brodie Creek Park, the Colman Creek Greenway, and Fourche Bottoms. They also hope to expand their network of trails into the city park properties located to the north across Fourche Creek. This area has been underused recently and contains scenic lakes and lots of paved trails.

If you want to get involved, search for "Meadowcliff Brookwood Neighborhood Association" on Facebook.

Little Rock Trail Network (Part of "A City in a Park")

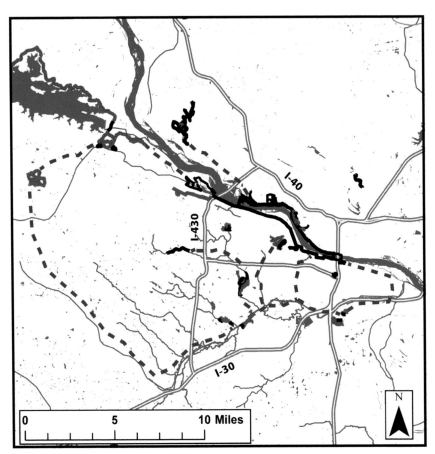

Little Rock's Parks Master Plan includes a series of connected trails surrounding and running through the city. The map shows how this could look in the near future. In some places a few short connecting pieces (see the area around UALR) could dramatically increase the continuous length of trails in the city and begin to allow these trails to serve as transportation routes in addition to being places to enjoy the outdoors. The River Trail already serves both functions as it connects major residential areas of Little Rock to job locations in North Little Rock and Downtown Little Rock.

Rose Creek Trail

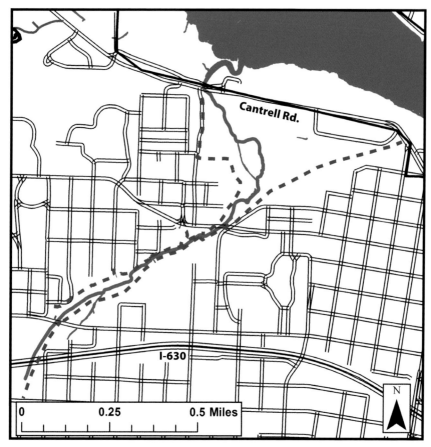

A trail along Rose Creek in the Capitol View, Stift Station neighborhoods was considered and partially planned many years ago. A renewed interest by the neighborhoods and city government in connecting the River Trail to these neighborhoods and perhaps all the way to Interstate 630 and Fourche Bottoms means this trail may soon become a reality. This trail would provide a safe and scenic way for people to commute by bike from these neighborhoods to downtown.

Other Resources:

Biking

Bicycle Advocacy of Central Arkansas (BACA) - http://www.bacar.org/

Bicycling in Arkansas Brochure (available at Burns Park and http://www.arkansas.com/outdoors/biking/)

River Trail Rentals – http://River Trailrentals.com

Hiking

Trails of Arkansas Blog: http://trailsofarkansas.blogspot.com/

Little Rock Parks - http://www.littlerock.org/parksrecreation/

North Little Rock Parks - http://www.nlrpr.org/

Tim Ernst Books: http://www.timernst.com/

Floating

Arkansas Canoe Club: http://arkansascanoeclub.com/

Ozark Outdoor Supply: http://ozarkoutdoor.com/

Saline River Canoe: http://salinerivercanoe.com

Locations mentioned in this book

Audubon Arkansas Nature Center: http://ar.audubon.org

Bell Slough: http://www.agfc.com

Fourche Creek: http://fourchecreek.org/

Lorance Creek: http://www.naturalheritage.com/natural-area/lorance-creek/

Maumelle River WMA: http://www.agfc.com

Pinnacle Mountain State Park:
http://www.arkansasstateparks.com/pinnaclemountain/

Ouachita Trail: http://www.friendsot.org

Toltec Mounds: http://www.arkansasstateparks.com/toltecmounds/

About the Author

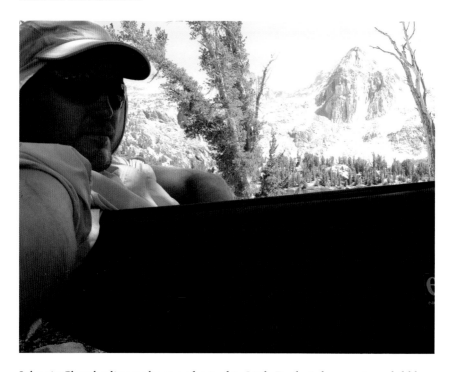

Johnnie Chamberlin was born and raised in Little Rock, Arkansas. As a child he often built dams in the creek near his backyard and frequently mucked around in other nearby drainage ditches despite being warned by his mother that they were contaminated with pesticides and rat poison. As he grew older, he managed to find new ways to pursue this love of splashing around in polluted waterways by researching bioremediation of Superfund sites in grad school, then studying and working on Fourche Creek in Little Rock, and finally by doing monitoring at oil spills in Michigan, Montana, and the Gulf of Mexico.

Johnnie is a Little Rock Central High graduate, has a BA in Cognitive Science from UC Berkeley, and a MS in Civil and Environmental Engineering from Duke University. He is currently working towards an Environmental Dynamics PhD at UA Fayetteville. He enjoys hiking, kayaking, swimming, biking, running, traveling all over and he tries to go on at least one backpacking trip a year.